Herbal
WELL-BEING

Simple Recipes for Making Your Own
Herbal Medicines, Aromatherapy Blends,
and Herbal Body-Care Formulas

Joyce A. Wardwell ❋ Colleen K. Dodt ❋ Greta Breedlove

D1354305

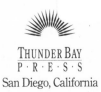

THUNDER BAY
P · R · E · S · S
San Diego, California

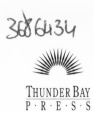

THUNDER BAY
P · R · E · S · S

Thunder Bay Press
An imprint of the Advantage Publishers Group
5880 Oberlin Drive, San Diego, CA 92121-4794
www.advantagebooksonline.com

Edited by Deborah Balmuth and Karen Levy
Original text design by Carol J. Jessop, Black Trout Design
Text production by Susan Bernier and Kelley Nesbit
Indexed by Eileen M. Clawson

ISBN 1-57145-813-1
Library of Congress Cataloging-in-Publication Data available upon request.

Printed in the United States by R.R. Donnelley
10 9 8 7 6 5 4 3 2 1

TABLE OF CONTENTS

INTRODUCTION

My great-grandmother Na never went to a doctor in her life. She dismissed the doctors as charlatans, saw their medicines as harmful, and thought hospitals were places you went to die. Her back-then attitudes weren't that much different from our attitudes today, only now we mistrust shifty HMOs, spiraling hospital bills, and the side effects of drugs. Just like my grandmother, we believe that "I can do it better." One of the most famous doctors of this century, Dr. Albert Schweitzer, expressed exactly this sentiment: "It's supposed to be a professional secret, but I'll tell you anyway. We doctors do nothing. We only help and encourage the doctor within."

Indeed, roughly 80 percent of the world's population uses herbal medicine for primary health care. And lest you doubt the effectiveness of plant remedies, realize that about 30 percent of prescription drugs are still synthesized from plants. In fact, the word *drug* comes from an old Dutch word, *drogge,* which means "to dry" — a reference to the preparation of medicinal plants, of course.

Na never went to a doctor, because she had her stock of home herbal remedies. She raised three healthy children plying her craft. But her fear and mistrust of doctors also had its downside. She spent the last thirty years of her life blind with cataracts and having to sit most of the time because she had a prolapsed uterus — two conditions that modern medicine could have easily remedied. Today, we are fortunate enough to have access to the best of both worlds: We can use traditional medicine and techniques to keep ourselves healthy and prevent ailments from becoming deadly; and we can turn to either modern or alternative medicine for treatment when the crisis is beyond our capability, skills, or equipment.

Twenty years ago, when I set out to learn about plants, teachers and practitioners of herbal medicine were few and far

CAUTION

Like any medicine, herbs should be used with care. The simple herbal recipes in this book are meant to inspire and are not given as medical advice. For your individual health concerns, for chronic warning symptoms, in emergency situations, or when in doubt, seek the advice of your primary personal health care practitioner.

between in the United States. Happily, I was able to meet up with healers from different traditions who each dropped a clue, gave a hint, or told a story to help me on my path. But always I found myself returning to the plants themselves as my teachers. Books and teachers tell you about the plants, but the better way to learn is to work with the plants, letting them tell you about themselves.

Looking back, the path I was left to take was a fortunate gift. I was forced to develop my own way of relating to herbs and medicine. I had to seek it myself.

This book is not meant to be a complete course in herbal medicine. It is, rather, a guide to help you walk your own medicine path. Inside you'll find suggestions, options, and exercises. There is no one best way to use herbs. But if you try the various techniques within, perhaps you'll discover the one best way that works for you.

With the creation of herbal treatments, a relationship as old as the beginning of time is also honored and renewed. This relationship with our green friends and the healing gifts they offer to us in the form of herbs, flowers, trees, and fragrances is a relationship offering peace. My hope and my wish for you is a greater connection first to yourself, then of course to others and this wonderful planet of ours. Green Blessings.

—*Joyce A. Wardwell*

PART I:
HERBAL HOME REMEDIES

Simple Recipes for Tinctures, Teas, Salves, Tonics, and Syrups

Joyce A. Wardwell

THE CHALLENGE OF HERBALISM:
SO MUCH TO LEARN

The *Wall Street Journal* now backs information as being more valuable than gold. The Internet has only increased our fear of being out of date. Every day there is so much more new information that we are hard pressed to keep up — it is the new stress for the new millennium. Indeed, the field of herbalism is a prime example. No one — even with a computer — can keep up with all the new information concerning plants and their medicinal attributes that is constantly developing or being brought to the forefront from modern research, the Amazon rain forests, the Ivory coast, ayurvedic medicine, Tibetan medicine, traditional Chinese medicine, and other means.

Great gobs of money are being spent trying to find patentable medicines and extracts to cure cancer, AIDS, leukemia, and even baldness — anything that people will spend great gobs of money to fix. In the past years I've seen feverfew change from a largely forgotten herb to one in the highest demand. Other fads will come and go: blue-green algae, wheat grass, *kombu-cha,* raw foods, and bee pollen, to name a few.

But the simple medicinal weeds in your backyard will always be there for you to use, without any multilevel marketing schemes, exorbitant price tags, dangerous side effects, exploitation of third-world child labor, expensive equipment, capital, or even fancy packaging to throw away. What do you think the people of post–World War II Germany turned to for medicine — encapsulated supplemental formulas, expensive Western pharmaceuticals, or tree bark? To this day Germany's reliance on herbal medicine sets the standard for the world. They learned firsthand to treasure their weeds. We can do the same.

CHAPTER 1

Stocking the Home Medicine Chest

Medicine is for the patient . . .
Medicine is for the people . . .
It is not for the profits.

— George Merck

Putting together an herbal first-aid medicine chest is a bit like playing the stock market. From a list of companies (the herbs) you choose a few to research and invest in (gathering and preparing), in the hopes that a profit will be made (health). Once one stock (herb) gives you a tidy profit, you are that much more likely to reinvest in it and perhaps expand to try another.

There will be losses, too. Every year I add to my compost pile some of the dried herbs I didn't need because no one broke a bone or had the flu. In fact, many people find that at first they use herbs mostly to treat a cold or earache — acute conditions. But as time goes by, and they start to rely on daily doses of nourishing and gentle herbs, they find that acute conditions happen less frequently, because bones are denser, immunity is stronger, and stress has reduced its hold.

LET NATURE BE YOUR HMO

Just as the stock market changes, so will your family's medicinal needs change. When my children were babies, I relied on big jars of gentle salves and herbs rich in nutrients. When they entered public school, cold prevention became a concern. When sports entered the picture, I stockpiled plants for sprains, cuts, and building stamina.

A good home medicine chest will take into account everyone's needs and have appropriate preparations on hand, ready to use when needed. Since some time and effort goes into this, remember it's also important to store the medicine chest in a cool dark place (and, always, out of the reach of small children) so the medicinals last as long as possible.

BASIC ELEMENTS OF THE HERBAL HOME MEDICINE CHEST

While there are specialty preparations you'll want to have hand-tailored to your family's particular health needs, there are a few standard elements that are useful to have in almost any herbal medicine chest.

ALL-PURPOSE SALVE

This should be a good all-purpose preparation that is antiseptic, speeds healing, and soothes inflamed tissues. Plantain, St.-John's-wort, lavender, thyme, poplar bark, and balsam poplar buds, or combinations thereof, are possible herbs to include in this salve.

ANTIVIRAL TINCTURE

When a virus runs through the house, it can take away everyone's energy — even for those who don't get the bug. I consider a good antiviral tincture or syrup indispensable and essential to have ready to use. St.-John's-wort, raw garlic, honey, red clover, and thyme are all good ingredients for helping the body's immune system ward off invading viruses.

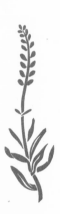

ASTRINGENT WASH

A mild astringent is handy for relieving mild sunburns, stanching bleeding from cuts, soothing insect bites, relieving swollen tissues, and cleansing the face. Dilute rose leaf tincture with 2 parts water and use as a wash; for a stronger action, use walnut leaf tincture.

BALSAM POPLAR BUD TINCTURE

To prevent tape burn, paint the skin with this tincture before applying tape or bandages.

BRUISE AND SPRAIN TREATMENT

Dried plantain leaf, lavender blossom, and poplar bark work well for treating these conditions. Make a tea and lay on the affected area in the form of a poultice to help speed healing and reduce inflammation.

COUGH AND COLD RELIEF

A jar of pine pitch is indispensable for these conditions — use it as a steam pot to break up congestion, or mix it in a salve with peppermint so it can be rubbed on the chest or on sore, aching muscles.

A few pieces of dried mallow root are also important to have; chewing on this root helps relieve a sore throat. You could also make peppermint-thyme cough drops, which simultaneously aid the body's immune system and soothe a sore throat. Add mullein, violet, poplar, or garlic to help break up congestion.

DISINFECTANT

Thyme, garlic, lavender, poplar bark, and white pine are all antiseptic by themselves. To disinfect cuts, wash with a tea made from one of these herbs, or make a rubbing alcohol tincture from the herb for a healing disinfectant.

HANGOVER RELIEF

Borage oil is useful for rebuilding the strength after a debilitating illness and as a quick remedy for a hangover taken along with a piece or two of candied ginger. (It also makes an excellent topical oil for dry, itchy skin.)

NAUSEA, INDIGESTION, AND MOTION SICKNESS RELIEF

These conditions can be alleviated by sucking on a few pieces of candied ginger, which is handy to have and stores for a considerable length of time. Also, peppermints or candies made from lavender or catnip may help.

PAIN RELIEF

It can be difficult to be always brewing up teas when in pain. Make a tincture or vinegar to have on hand. Lavender and poplar bark are good for general pain relief. Lemon balm, catnip, and oat straw add a calming dimension as well. Use internally or externally as needed.

FACTORS AFFECTING WHAT'S IN YOUR FAMILY'S MEDICINE CHEST

Ages of members
Personal health needs
Personal goals and temperaments
Lifestyle demands
Access to herbs
Travel requirements and interests

SALVE FOR CUTS, SCRAPES, WOUNDS, AND BURNS

When I need more than a simple salve, I turn to white pine pitch — the original liquid Band-Aid. Though it will collect dirt on top, the pitch makes an airtight bandage that is antiseptic underneath. Cover it with a piece of tissue to keep it from sticking to everything. As long as there is no infection, do not remove old

THE MINIMALIST'S MEDICINE CHEST

Herbs can do double and triple duty in your herbal medicine chest. If your resources are limited, choose just one or two multipurpose herbs to begin building your chest: ginger, lavender, peppermint, plantain, poplar, and white pine are all good choices. Each has a wide variety of applications for acute and crisis conditions.

Plantain is my own personal favorite, and it doesn't cost me a cent. When I moved to a place that had no plantain growing nearby, I asked a local market farmer if I could take some plantain from his fields. He was sure I was certifiable, but he even dug and potted the plants for me! But which is crazier: refusing to see the value in what lies under your feet, or purposefully planting weeds in a garden?

I planted the plantain within 10 feet of my door, where it provides a strong contrasting backdrop for my colorful Johnny-jump-ups. Sure, it spreads quickly, but no faster than I use it for medicine and food. So nine months of the year, a valued component of my herbal medicine chest lies right by my doorstep. The other three months, I dig up about a dozen plants and plant them closely in a 2-gallon pot with average soil. Plantain thrives on neglect, but not on poor drainage, so add some sand if your soil has a lot of clay in it. The pot stays by a sunny window through the winter — offering me a year-round supply.

I use plantain much in the way you might an aloe, for poultices for sprains and relief from cuts, mild burns, and swellings. It can be used freely because nature renews the supply, come spring. Plantain happens to be my standard all-purpose remedy. Other people swear by lavender, comfrey, heal-all, nettle, or another plant. Whatever herb you choose is fine; just be sure you have it handy year-round.

pitch; instead, keep applying new fresh pitch until the cut is healed. A salve made from balsam poplar buds will have similar qualities and is good if your skin is sensitive to white pine pitch.

STYPTIC
For bleeding from razor cuts, keep some powdered peppermint leaf on hand — just a sprinkle will stop the bleeding.

Equipment and Supplies

In addition to the herbs and preparations, you'll need the following supplies for applying and administering them and performing other first-aid duties:

- A glass dropper that can squirt either a few drops of tincture under a tongue or a few drops of healing oil into a sore ear
- An atomizer for spraying herb teas on the back of sore throats, over large areas of skin, or up stuffy noses
- An Ace bandage to apply loosely for keeping a poultice in place, or tighter for supporting a sprained limb
- Fine needle for removing splinters
- A sharp razor for removing hair around cuts
- Clean lengths of muslin or gauze in a couple of different sizes for use as handcloths to wash areas with herb teas, or (in larger sizes) to make poultices to lay on the affected area
- First-aid tape
- Tissues
- Pieces of gauze
- Cotton swabs
- Tweezers
- Small sharp scissors

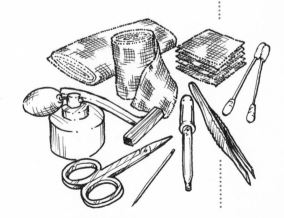

A Jar of Honey

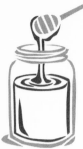

A jar of honey is another valuable first-aid readiness tool to have in the house. A medicine in its own right, honey has powerful antibacterial properties. Pure honey literally sucks the moisture out of bacteria, effectively killing them, while leaving you un-harmed. Applied straight it heals external ulcers, wounds, cold sores, genital herpes sores, cysts, and other stubborn-healing sores. Taken internally, it soothes the gastrointestinal tract, calms nerves and spasms, gives energy, and helps the body maintain a stable electrolyte balance (critical when diarrhea, vomiting, or fevers are present). Honey also increases the med-icinal effect of natural remedies — especially for the respiratory system. Simply add the indicated medicinal herb dose to a cup of warm water sweetened with honey and sip frequently.

Another technique is to blend equal amounts of honey and herb tincture and use this mixture as needed. Or, mix equal amounts of the freshly chopped herb and honey, let rest for twenty minutes, then apply as needed.

A Beneficial Supply of Yogurt

When illness threatens, stock up on plain yogurt. The beneficial bacteria in yogurt keep the body's digestive system working at peak efficiency. (*Note:* These bacteria are destroyed when sugar or fruit are added, so for medicinal purposes, use only plain yogurt.) Spastic stomachs can usually keep a teaspoon of yogurt down, and that teaspoon will help restore the stomach to a calm condition. A cup of yogurt added to a bath will soothe bladder and vaginal yeast infections, as will a douche made with 2 tablespoons of yogurt in a quart of warm water.

If you must embark on a course of antibiotic treatment, eat a cup of yogurt every day during and for several weeks after treatment. Antibiotics indiscriminately destroy both harmful and necessary bacteria in the body. Eating yogurt reintroduces into the digestive tract beneficial bacteria — the ones without which the digestive process cannot function. Eating plain yogurt will also help prevent renegade yeasts such as candida from multiplying to harmful levels (this is why vaginal yeast infections are so common after a course of antibiotics).

CHAPTER 2
Selecting Quality
Ingredients and Equipment

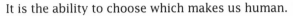

It is the ability to choose which makes us human.

— Madelaine L'Engle, *Walking on Water:*
Reflections on Faith and Art

An herb's quality determines its healing capacity. Would you eat a salad made from brown wilted lettuce or dried lettuce greens? Certainly not by choice. If it were served in a restaurant you'd demand a refund. Yet we pay for poor-quality herbs wrapped in expensive high-quality packages all the time. To ensure that we have the best herbal medicine, we must train ourselves to look beyond the wrapping and into the herb itself.

WHAT MAKES A QUALITY HERB?

Given all possible choices, I *always* choose the fresh herb. The fresh plant has a vitality that quickly degrades. Studies done by the Rodale Institute show that a head of broccoli left out in the sun can lose as much as half of its vitamin C content in the first half hour! In the refrigerator, nutrient loss slows but still occurs. Careful herbalists gather or grow their own herbs whenever possible to ensure the best quality.

Dried Herbs: Read the Labels

If fresh herbs are unavailable, use dried herbs or products made from certified organic herbs. First try your local county extension office to see who may be growing and selling organic herbs in your area. Or, to purchase retail, look for products stamped with a label from one of the following organic associations whose members have taken a pledge to uphold certain voluntary standards: The Organic Crop Improvement Association (OCIA), Farm-verified Organics, Organic Buyers and Growers Association (OBGA), or the California Certification for Organic Farmers, the latter being regulated by the California state government. As of this writing, there are no *national* guidelines for organic certification, and because of strife between organic growers and the United States Department of Agriculture, there may never be such guidelines.

There are not even any voluntary controls on imported herbs. Pesticides such as DDT that are banned in the United States are routinely used in other nations. In addition, imported herbs must be warehoused for extended periods of time and are routinely fumigated with a toxic soup of chemicals to prevent mold, fungal growth, and insect infestations. Now imagine taking these imported herbs as medicine . . . no thanks. Be particular: About 75 percent of botanicals in medicinal products are imported. Of the remaining 25 percent grown domestically, only a small percentage are certified as organically grown.

Once I find that an herb is certified organic (or ethically wildcrafted) I check the label for a date. Most dried herbs have a shelf life of one year, although some with fleeting essences, such as lemon balm, are only medicinally viable for about six months. Commercial vinegared herbs are considered potent for about one year; tinctures and glycerates for about five years in optimal storage conditions. Heat, light, and air all degrade the quality of the herb. Herbs displayed in clear glass jars in a sunny window have their medicinal virtues compromised. Don't buy them.

> I believe a leaf of grass
> is no less
> Than the journey work
> of the stars.
>
> — Walt Whitman,
> "Song of Myself"

Rely on Your Senses!

If there is no date on the package of dried herbs you're buying — and usually there isn't — take a close look at the herb. The color should be deep and rich, comparable to its living color. Smell it; the odor should be full and strong. The herb itself should be crisp and dry. If you're buying an herb cream, tincture, oil, or other mixture, make sure there is no separation, precipitate, or surface mold. All of these are signs of poor manufacturing or storage.

Be Suspicious of Capsules

Ever notice how you can't check the quality of herb capsules until after you buy them? To test the quality, pour the contents of a purchased herb capsule into a bowl and a bit of a similar dried herb into another bowl for comparison. The whole dried herb will have a stronger smell and color, indicative of a higher quality herb. That's because capsules generally contain the worst-quality herbs commercially available. And even if the manufacturer purchases high-quality herbs to make the capsules, it honestly doesn't matter. The encapsulation process itself ruins the herb.

Have you ever shredded lettuce and let it sit for a couple of hours? It soon wilts, then rots quickly. When an herb is pulverized into powder, the heat generated by the equipment literally cooks the herb. Decay accelerates because more of the herb is exposed to air. Then the encapsulated powder sits decaying further on a shelf for months or years before it's purchased.

When finally ingested, a capsule can take thirty minutes to dissolve, completely bypassing the stomach's digestion and relying on the small intestine for initial breakdown (not the small intestine's best function). You'd probably get a greater medicinal value by making a cup of tea from a first-cutting hay bale. A cup of tea made from hay will start to enter the bloodstream before you even swallow. Hay certainly costs a lot less and is usually locally available. And most farmers won't spray a hayfield, since it's not cost-effective. But don't go out and start using hay for medicine — there is one important piece of information about a hay bale you don't know: what plants are inside. The risk of toxic herbs being present is just too great!

Using capsules can give us an herb, but it can never nurture our spirits the way other methods of herb use do. Taking the time to sip a cup of tea or to soak in an herb bath reaffirms the healing process. It helps to slow your pace, empower your being, and delight your senses.

MAKING YOUR OWN CAPSULES

If you have to have your herbs in capsule form for convenience's sake, it's best to make your own. This is best done by grinding the herb by hand with a mortar and pestle, since a mechanical grinder generates too much heat. Make only one or two days' supply at a time, and refrigerate the capsules until used.

GOOD MEDICINE STARTS WITH
GOOD INGREDIENTS

In addition to herbs, there are a number of other ingredients we are going to need for creating our own homemade remedies. As a self-reliant herbalist, I want these additional ingredients to be of as high a quality as the herbs I use. Let the large mass-manufacturer of lip balm use less expensive paraffin wax instead of beeswax. For my purposes, the extra half penny per ounce that beeswax costs is well worth the difference on my baby's chapped bottom.

A Guide to Quality

There are several basic ingredients you'll be using over and over again for the recipes in this book. Following is a description of these ingredients, along with advice on how to ensure purity and the highest quality for each.

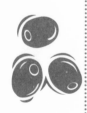

OILS

Oils exposed to light and heat quickly become rancid, and rancid oils are carcinogenic. If an oil is in a clear bottle, glass or plastic, it may well be rancid. It's important to ask the store owner how long the oil has been sitting on the shelf. An owner who is confident about the quality of the oils may let you sample. One quick way to test for rancidity is to put a drop of oil on the back of your tongue: If it burns, it is rancid. Another good policy is to purchase medicinal oils that are packaged in tins or dark bottles. Be sure that any oils you buy are cold-pressed; any other extraction process uses chemical solvents to increase the oil yield.

Internal use. My oil of choice for internal consumption is olive oil. It is readily available in tins, is quality graded, and tastes delicious. Olive oil is also rich in antioxidants, which are food compounds (such as the vitamins A, C, and E and carotenes and selenium) that combat destructive free oxygen molecules. Antioxidants thus help the body fight degenerative and age-related illnesses. Adding an herb such as ginger to the olive oil allows it to do double duty as a healing oil and a base for cooking, saving a little work. When colds are coming on in our family, I will often sauté a little ginger root or other warming herb in the olive oil I am using to make dinner. That way we can have our medicine and eat it too.

In selecting olive oil, you should know that it is graded: The first cold-pressing yields the highest grade, extra virgin, which is best for internal uses. Organically grown cold-pressed canola oil makes a less expensive substitute. When I'm on a budget, I mix equal amounts of olive oil and canola oil, with satisfactory results.

External use (absorption). As an external absorption oil used to soften, moisturize, and maintain healthy skin, I prefer to use jojoba oil (which technically is a plant ester, not an oil). It is readily absorbed by the skin and resists rancidity. It is priced competitively with other absorbing oils such as sesame, walnut, wheat germ, and safflower. Unlike these oils, however, jojoba oil should not be used internally.

External use (nonabsorbent). For a nonabsorbent oil (for massages, chapped skin, diaper rash), use one that forms a protective barrier on the skin. Oils that are not absorbed as easily and are pleasant to work with include sweet almond, virgin olive, avocado, peanut, apricot kernel, and cocoa butter.

ALCOHOLS

Alcohols are primarily used to make tinctures. The concentration of alcohol is usually expressed as a percentage; multiply the percentage by 2 to get what is called the proof. Thus 80-proof vodka is 40 percent alcohol. Any 80-proof alcohol will make an acceptable tincture for most herbs. If 190-proof (95 percent alcohol, also known as everclear or grain alcohol) is legally available in your area, I recommend using it instead. Using 190-proof offers several advantages over lower-proof alcohol:

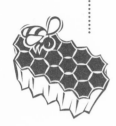

- ◆ Less is required per dose.
- ◆ With grain alcohol I can easily control the amount of water I add. The alcohol extracts the herb by desiccation, essentially wringing out the aromatic essences of the herb into the alcohol. Some herbs, such as ginger, need the stronger concentration of alcohol because some of their medicinal compounds are not fully solvent in water. Some herbs (most flowers and leaves) need more water.
- ◆ It has a longer shelf life.
- ◆ Because of the further distillation, the alcohol is less likely to have wayside contaminants or flavoring agents added.

WINES

Don't use commercial wines for medicine making. Wine grapes are heavily sprayed with fungal and mold inhibitors, and sulfites and cadmium are used to make the wine. Studies have also shown that the foil wrapper around the seal leaks lead into the wine. But don't rule out medicinal wines altogether; Chapter 6 includes recipes for simple, low-cost medicinal wines you can make at home.

VINEGARS

A good-quality vinegar is alive. Vinegar is made by inoculating wine with bacteria (called the mother vinegar). A living vinegar is slightly cloudy, and there is a sediment on the bottom of the bottle. You can buy apple cider vinegar with the mother in it at most health food stores, but it is a bit pricey. Chapter 6 includes instructions for making your own vinegar for a few pennies a gallon.

GLYCERIN

Glycerin is used to make tinctures for children or adults who wish to avoid alcohol. Glycerin's sweetness helps mask unpleasant flavors. Use a 100-percent-vegetable-based glycerin; the quality is higher than animal-based glycerin and is safe for human consumption. The shelf life is comparable to that of alcohol tinctures, though glycerin does not extract resins or oils from plants well.

Glycerin should be diluted with water when making the tincture (the same as alcohol, but remember, many alcohols are purchased diluted). Use pure distilled water to ensure no wayside contaminants. A tincture made with glycerin is called a glycerate. Excessive consumption of glycerate tinctures may cause diarrhea in sensitive individuals. (See page 41 for standard tincture doses.)

HONEY

Buy honey that is free of pesticides and contaminants. By and large I find that small beekeepers avoid using sprays — perhaps because beekeeping by its very nature involves an understanding of nature's web. Try to buy honey grown close to your home. Each country — indeed, each county — produces a distinct type of honey. People with hay fever or allergies sometimes find relief from eating local honey. Stop at your local farmer's market, and find a person who is selling crystallized honey. This honey is raw and unfiltered. Raw honey contains enzymes that have antibiotic abilities — enzymes that are destroyed by light and heat, making raw honey the best choice for medicinal use. I think it tastes better as well. There are people who swear by the superior qualities of dark honey; however, medicinally I find little difference between the two.

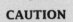

CAUTION

The Centers for Disease Control in Atlanta recommends that raw honey should not be given to children under one year old. You may wish to play it safe and avoid giving honey to children for their first two years. Some uncooked honeys may contain botulism spores that are harmless for the older child and adult, but can cause a fatal diarrhea in an immature digestive system.

BEESWAX

Try to buy your beeswax from a local beekeeper. You'll get a better-quality wax for a much lower price. The beekeeper I get wax from charges me $6 per pound; the local craft store charges $2.50 per ounce! Don't worry if there are a few bee wings or such in the wax. Wax acts as a preservative, and you can simply strain out the stray pieces when you melt it.

SUGARS

Sugars are used to make wines and syrups, and to sweeten bitter brews. Alternatives to refined white table sugar include honey (see previous) and maple syrup. Maple syrup contains trace minerals that are carried up in a tree's sap from as much as 60 feet below the ground. A pure maple syrup has a flowery aroma and buttery texture. Grade A Amber syrup comes from the first flow of sap and is considered the best.

Stevia. This herbal sweetener has been used worldwide for centuries, but has been available in the United States only since 1988. The Food and Drug Administration has not approved stevia as a sweetener, only as a food additive. It's up to three hundred times sweeter than sugar; use just 1 teaspoon of stevia in place of 1 cup of sugar. Its sweetening ability is similar to that of sucrose, with little aftertaste. Stevia has a fleeting flavor, reminiscent of honeysuckle, that seems to disappear in tea or cooking. Another plus is that stevia is not a nutrition source for oral bacteria; it actually helps suppress cavities!

SALTS

Salts are effective for preserving herbs to be used in baths. Common table salt, sodium chloride, is generally not recommended, but will do if no other salt is available. Sea salt, refined from ocean brine and rich in minerals, is my preference. Epsom salt, also known as magnesium sulfate, is an inexpensive alternative when you're making bath salts.

BASIC EQUIPMENT: AS CLOSE AS YOUR KITCHEN

The equipment you use to make your remedies will affect how they turn out. The good news is that home herbalism requires no special distillers, tubes, condensers, or other supplies. Chances are you have everything you need already — or you can find it at a garage sale for next to nothing.

NOTEBOOK

A blank notebook is your most important piece of equipment. Be sure to keep track of your favorite recipes, references, and suppliers' addresses and telephone numbers. Because I gather or grow nearly all my herbs, I also note the seasonal and daily weather conditions, gathering dates and places. I write notes and observations about the preparation process. I even write down my mistakes — they are valuable little lessons that I don't wish to repeat.

LABELS

However large or small, fancy or plain, labels are the herbalist's best friend. Use them relentlessly; a remedy is not finished until it has a label on it. At the very least, list the ingredients and the date. Other helpful items to list are: what the preparation is for, how it should be used, how it should be stored, and where the herbs were obtained.

GLASS JARS

Colored glass jars and bottles with lids are trea-
sures to any herbalist. Check out your
local recycling station for free jars. A
local restaurant-bar lets me haul
away as many empty liquor and
wine bottles and 1-gallon-
size pickle jars as I care to —
Saturday night offers me the
best selection. Second-hand
shops always offer interesting
selections, usually for less than a
dime apiece. Disinfect the bottles
before using by boiling for 10 min-
utes, or rinse with a 3 percent hydrogen peroxide solution, commonly available at a grocery store or pharmacy. Simply wash

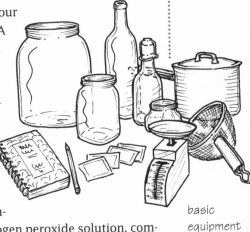

basic
equipment

your jars with soap and water and rinse. Then, pour a small amount of peroxide into the jar, shake vigorously, and drain. Last, rinse with water and air dry.

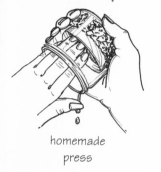

homemade
press

STRAINER AND PRESS

To strain a cup of tea, any stainless-steel sieve works well. But you might notice that, when you strain, you're losing a lot of precious liquid from the loose herbs — that's valuable medicine. Likewise, when we talk about casually tossing out the spent herbs used to make a jojoba herb oil or a carefully compiled tincture, suddenly every drop that can be pressed from them becomes precious. A press works much better than a strainer for these purposes.

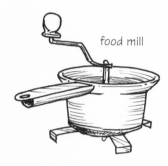

food mill

A quick and effective homemade press can be assembled simply from a lid that fits inside your jar. Apply wrist pressure to the lid to squeeze out as much liquid extract as possible. I have used a food mill (the kind used to strain baby food) with more satisfying results. But for the best extraction, it is hard to beat a wine press. This piece of equipment is common, inexpensive, and easy to use. You can find one at most kitchen accessory stores or beer and wine-making suppliers. Do tell them that you are using it only for home herb use lest they try to sell you a commercial grape crusher!

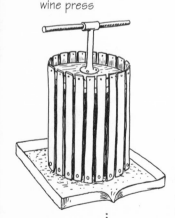

wine press

MORTAR AND PESTLE

If you're only going to buy one piece of special equipment for making herbal remedies, this is it. A mortar and pestle for grinding dried roots, leaves, and seeds is the only way to be assured of a fresh herb powder. A traditional European mortar has smooth sides. A Japanese mortar, called a *suribachi,* has grooves and ridges on the sides; I find this style to be more efficient. If you live near a flowing creek, you can look to any little waterfalls for natural stone mortars made of quartz or basalt. I have a 2-foot stone slab that I use as my mortar, along with fist-size round rocks for my pestles for extra-quick grinding.

Herbs can also be ground efficiently in a hand-cranked coffee grinder set aside just for herbs. (Don't use it to grind coffee afterward, or your coffee will taste like the herbs.) And even though electric coffee grinders may seem more efficient, try to avoid them. The herbs get too hot, which destroys delicate oils and essences. If you need the ease of an electric grinder, some experienced medicine makers freeze the herbs first to keep temperatures to a minimum. Grind small batches using only short bursts and you can keep the herbs from getting hot.

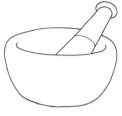

mortar and pestle

SAUCEPAN

Reserve one 1- or 2-quart pan just for making salves. Oils and beeswax leave hard-to-clean residues behind in the pan. It only took one batch of waxy chicken soup to convince me that a separate salve pan was a wise investment. Similarly, reserve one stainless steel or birch stirring spoon and one stainless-steel mesh strainer that fits over your saucepan for salve making.

SCALE

A small diet scale is a useful piece of equipment to have on hand for making herbal remedies, since weight is a more precise unit of measure than volume. For most mild herbs, the medicinal dose is 1 ounce of herb to 32 ounces of water. Because an ounce of dried leaves has greater volume than an ounce of root, most beginners find it helpful to use a scale until they become accustomed to the proportions.

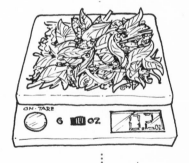

scale

However, I never did use a scale for making medicine with mild herbs until I began to teach others. I reasoned that since the herbs were relatively safe, exploring the differences in taste and potency was more important to me than obtaining a precise measurement. And since an herb's relative strength depends on so many variables, it isn't possible to measure potency anyway — unless you have equipment far more sophisticated than a simple scale. Still, when you're starting out, a scale will help you get a feel for the relative suggested proportions.

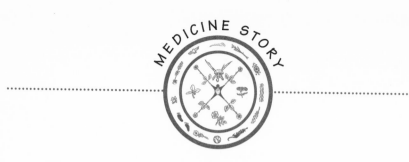

MEDICINE STORY

HOW TO FIND A LOST ARROW — OR ANYTHING ELSE

One day a young Native American boy was playing with his toy arrows, and one by one broke all of them. He wanted to keep playing, so he went and took one of his father's arrows. Now, all a man owns is his bow and arrows and clothes; everything else — the wigwam, the skins, the food, even the children — belongs to the women. Each man's arrows are treasured and many hours are spent crafting them and making them perfect. They protect, provide his people with meat, and give him honor. This boy must have been young indeed not to remember this when he took his father's arrow.

All the boy knew was how well his shots flew — farther and faster than ever. Once, the arrow went so far that he lost sight of it. But he was able to mark the arrow's flight and ran over to seek it in the place he had spotted. To his dismay, the area was a muddy overgrown tangle. He climbed a nearby tree to peer in, but he couldn't see the arrow anywhere. So he plunged into the thicket to look. He knew he'd better find that arrow!

His first steps covered his moccasins with mud. He searched and he searched, but he couldn't find the arrow. He kept worrying about what his father would say or do to him, until he made himself scared. He looked till he was tired, and hot, and frustrated. It wasn't until he felt itchy all over that he finally noticed where he really was — right in the middle of a poison ivy patch! Now he was in big trouble! His father was going to be furious, and his mother, too! No one could help him. Overwhelmed, the boy sat down and began to bawl.

Through his tears, he noticed a frog jump near his feet. "You're in big trouble too, frog," he said out loud. "Don't you know you'll get poison ivy all over your smooth skin, just like me?" The frog stared at him, jumped over to some broad-leafed plants, and rubbed his body against the leaves. Then he stuck out his tongue and jumped away.

So the boy gathered up some of those same leaves and rubbed himself, too. And as he stooped down to gather some more, he saw his father's arrow under the leaves. He picked it up and cleaned off the mud. He left behind a pinch of tobacco to thank the frog — and, I'm told, he even remembered to clean his moccasins!

Versions of this story are common among the Anishinaabe peoples of the northern Great Lakes region. The plant used in the story could be plantain, curly dock, or jewelweed. All grow near poison ivy, and each is effective against it.

CHAPTER 3
Making a Simple Cup of Tea

Simplicity is the final flower; behind it are cataclysms
of the soul and accumulations of wisdom,
just as behind the simplicity of a leaf are cosmic
and geological changes without number.

— Claude Bragdon, *The New Image*, 1928

Ever since some ingenious cavewoman threw a handful of wild herbs in her family's water-skin to keep the water tasting fresh and wholesome, herbal medicine has been with us — arguably the world's oldest science. Every single culture in the world steeps herbs in water for refreshing and medicinal drinks. Every single one.

Herbal medicine seems amazingly complex at first. There are over ten thousand plants listed in the collective written worldwide pharmacopeias! But just as nature has the salmon lay ten thousand eggs so that one might survive to adulthood, she has given us ten thousand plants to ensure that one will be available when we need it. A question I am often asked is, "What herb shall I take for my illness?" I like to answer, "Take any herb — just be sure it's a simple one!"

It's best to pick one or two plants that you are already familiar with and explore them fully. Only after you gain confidence in using those plants in teas, poultices, salves, or tinctures should you move on to learn about another plant. Let yourself build a basic foundation of knowledge from which one day you'll feel confident enough to dive into the whole pool of herbal medicine.

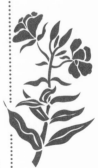

THE ART OF SIMPLING

Herbal medicine can be so easy that it's simple. In fact, it's even called simpling. But don't let the name fool you into thinking that simpling isn't as effective as more complex formulas. On

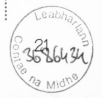

the contrary, simpling is the recommended course of treatment for most common acute ailments.

Four Elements

Successful simpling involves four elements or principles. First, you must use mild plants. These are often the plants commonly used as foods. They are safe enough for small children and the elderly, enhance the body's capacity to heal itself, and help create long-term health.

Second, you must use these mild herbs in large doses. The cup of tea you make from a paper tea bag may taste nice, but its medicinal action is negligible. Simpling involves making a strong pot of tea and drinking it several times throughout the day — for days, weeks, and sometimes months until a satisfactory cure is seen. For some chronic illnesses, such as diabetes, the simple herbs may become a lifelong habit.

The third element of simpling is that you must use herbs that grow nearby. The practical reason for this is purely economic. At three to ten dollars per ounce, you could easily spend upward of three hundred dollars a month for an herbal remedy. But more important, herbs take on the characteristics of their habitat. Just as herbs growing in wet places swell with water and therefore work better for kidney and bladder ailments, so herbs growing in cold climates tend to be more building and warming, and herbs grown in hot climates tend to be more eliminating and cooling.

To a certain extent, each climate tends to breed particular types of ailments in the people who live there. It is no surprise that you find more parasitic diseases in hotter climates, and more respiratory ailments in colder climates. By using the plants that grow in your own region, you are turning to the herbs that are best adapted for the stresses your climate puts on your body.

The fourth, and most important, element of simpling is that you must be patiently committed to following the course of the cure. It takes time to gather

FOUR ELEMENTS OF SIMPLING

1. Use mild herbs.
2. Use the herbs in large doses.
3. Use herbs that grow in or near the area where you live.
4. Be patient and committed to waiting for the effects of the tea you make.

herbs and make a simple tea, and it takes responsibility to drink that tea for several days or weeks as required. Usually, however, you should see some measure of relief within two to three days. If not, consider trying a different herb. When you use an herb for an extended period of time, take a rest from it one or two days a week, to give your body a chance to regain equilibrium.

For true healing to begin, you must also address other factors affecting health, such as stress, poor diet, exposure to toxins, and emotional or spiritual discontent. Lao-tzu said it well in his *Tao Te Ching:* "A person will get well only when he is tired of being sick."

HOW TO MAKE A SIMPLE TEA

The purpose of making a cup of tea is to extract the medicinal virtues of an herb into a cup of water. If you keep that in mind, the process becomes easy, and terms such as *decoction, infusion* (which are preparation techniques), *poultice, plaster,* and *fomentation* (application techniques) become unimportant. As you gain experience working with the herbs, methods of process and application do become important. But don't get hung up on definitions so much that you prevent yourself from exploring the herbs in the first place. Remember the intent is simply to make a cup of tea; the rest will follow.

The Method for Delicate Leaves and Flowers

Begin with 1 ounce of dried herb or 2 ounces of fresh herb; bring 1 quart of water to just under the boiling point, and pour it over the herb. Let steep for about 20 minutes, or until the water has absorbed the fragrance and color of the herb. This recipe will yield about 3 cups, which is one day's dose, taken ½ cup at a time through the day.

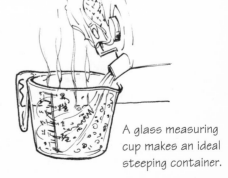

A glass measuring cup makes an ideal steeping container.

Alternate method. Another common method of simpling with flowers and leaves is to put the herb in cold water and let it steep in the sun for several hours. You can also put the herb in cold water and let it steep for 24 hours in the refrigerator. This method is preferred for herbs that have heat-sensitive volatile oils you want to preserve, such as mint and rose petal. It usually extracts the greatest amount of minerals from the herbs, but a lesser amount of tannins (which give herbs such as rose petal and blackberry their astringency).

The Method for Hardy Roots, Seeds, and Barks

It takes more effort to chew a root than to chew a leaf, and it takes more energy to extract the virtues from roots, seeds, and barks than from leaves or flowers. Grind, mash, or cut the herb first so as to expose more of its surface area to the water, making the extraction process more complete.

Measure 1 ounce of dried herb or 2 ounces fresh herb and combine in a saucepan with 1 quart of water. Simmer over low heat for 20 minutes to 1 hour. Herbs with important volatile oils, such as burdock, ginger, and mullein root, should be kept covered. For herbs left uncovered, a simple guideline is to simmer until the water is reduced by about one-third. This recipe yields 1 to 2 cups of tea, the daily dose, which is best drunk in small sips throughout the day.

Alternate method. Another method I like is making a sun tea. Begin by pouring 1 quart of boiling water over the cut or chopped herb. Put out in the sun and allow to sit for a full day. This process generally extracts less of an herb's medicinal attributes but keeps more of its vitamins and nutritive integrity.

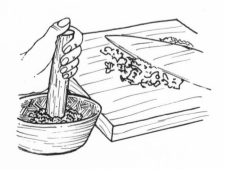

Mash or chop the hardy roots, seeds, and barks of herbs to prepare them for making tea.

SELECTING HERBS: START WITH WHAT YOU KNOW

As Maria Von Trapp said, "It's always best to start at the beginning." Look about you. What plants are you familiar with? Can you recognize a dandelion? A white pine tree? A strawberry? Now ask yourself what you have access to and make a list. These are the plants you should choose from for your teas. Just be sure to research the herb's safeness for consumption before you begin gathering.

Using Different Parts of the Plant

One of the gifts of herbalism is that one plant can yield us many medicines, depending on which part of the plant is used. As you work with an herb, explore its different parts. We know the strawberry best for its delicious fruit. However, the leaves, blossoms, stems, and roots all have valuable and different medicinal virtues — which vary further depending on when you gather them. Again, research the plant before you use it. For example, while rhubarb stalks are edible, rhubarb leaves can be poisonous. In the list that follows, you will find details about which parts of 25 plants are most commonly used.

TWENTY-FIVE SIMPLE HERBS
TO KNOW AND USE

The plants described on the following pages are a selection of perennial favorites for beginning students of herbalism. They are common, easy to recognize and gather, safe, and fun to work with. I encourage you to branch out and explore other plants as well.

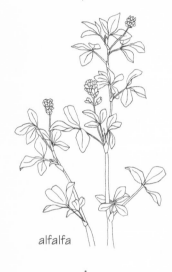

alfalfa

ALFALFA *(MEDICAGO SATIVA)*
The Arabic word for *alfalfa* means "father," and the plant was once reserved for warriors and prized horses. It's a superlative restorative tonic. Use the whole flowering plant for digestive weakness, for chronic inflammations, and to rebuild vitality. Deep taproots enable alfalfa to bring many trace minerals into its leaves, as well as vitamins C, D, E, and K. Though the roots aren't often used, I find that they make an excellent wash for chronic skin disorders.

BLACKBERRY (*RUBUS* SPP.)
To find the best stands of blackberry, look for their showy flowers in the spring. Blackberry root combats the deadly dysentery that runs rampant in close-quartered camps. In the American

ONE PERSON'S MEAT IS ANOTHER PERSON'S POISON

When trying a new plant, there is always the possibility of individual allergic reaction. Simple and mild herbs generally are safe to test at home. First, rub a bit of the plant on a patch of skin. If no swelling or itching occurs in 24 hours, try drinking a small amount of tea made from that herb. Wait 24 hours before taking a larger dose.

Some people find themselves allergic to many members of a whole family of plants. For example, people who are allergic to strawberry may have a similar reaction to rose hips or raspberry; all are members of the rose family of plants.

Revolutionary War, both sides accepted truces to enable the troops to "go rooting." The leaves are milder. Blackberry root (use for adults) or leaves (use for children) is still one of the safest and surest remedies for diarrhea. I make a blackberry root vinegar that excels at alleviating diarrhea caused both by flu or mild food poisoning. The flowers have a gentle sweetness that add a pleasant dimension to tea blends. And, of course, the fruits aren't so bad either.

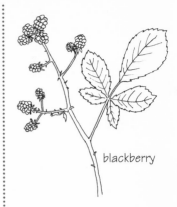

blackberry

BORAGE *(BORAGO OFFICINALIS)*
I only had to plant borage once — it volunteered thereafter. Borage's delicate blue flowers make salads and teas festive; they can also be added to homemade wine. The leaf, which has a cooling cucumber flavor, reduces fevers and calms irritated tissues. A glass of cold borage lemonade is one of the most refreshing summer drinks I know of; served hot it soothes a sore throat. The newly emerging leaves are a pleasant nibble, but as they grow they quickly get too prickly to eat. Having been a nursing mother of twins, I can assure you that borage ensures even milk production and high energy levels. Throughout history, borage has helped invalids regain their strength, and it works just as well today.

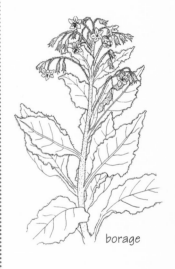

borage

The seed oil extract improves adrenal function, easing the stresses of menopause, obesity, rheumatism, and steroid or antibiotic treatments.

BURDOCK *(ARCTIUM LAPPA)*
Nature's Velcro and the original dart, burdock is one of the best tonic herbs — bar none. Use all parts; the seed and root are the most effective, however. Use the seeds externally for skin eruptions, while simultaneously using the root internally to treat the cause.

Burdock is used to eliminate toxins in the body. The root promotes sweating, increases

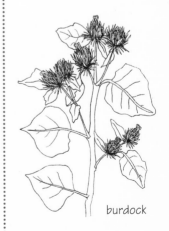

burdock

urine output, enhances liver function, and tastes very good in stir-fries, or slow-roasted or grilled. The peeled first-year stalk is another yummy food, similar to celery. The seeds are antibacterial and anti-inflammatory.

CATNIP *(NEPETA CATARIA)*

One of my first herbs of choice for children, nursing mothers, and the elderly, catnip calms the nerves, soothes digestion, and lowers a fever without raising it first. I've also used it successfully to ease colic, calm gastric and duodenal ulcers, aid digestion, increase milk flow, ease stress, and torment my cat.

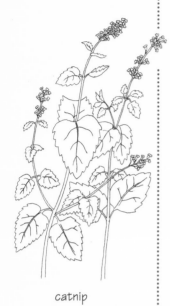

catnip

DANDELION *(TARAXACUM OFFICINALE)*

If you think you've never used dandelion as medicine, guess again. It's a prime ingredient in over half of all herb blends on the market, including formulas for weight loss, PMS, detoxification, and rejuvenation along with liver, digestive, kidney, and skin ailments! Dandelion is such a wondrous source of minerals, vitamins, fiber, micronutrients, lecithin, and biologically active substances that there is probably no existing condition that would not benefit from regularly consuming dandelions.

The greatest gift of dandelion is its safety record. Dandelion has no known cautionary drug interactions, cumulative toxic effects, or contraindications for use. This is one herb to allow yourself the full range of freedom to explore!

All parts are edible. The flowers make pleasant tea and wine, fritters and seasoning. The root can be steamed, broiled, roasted, and toasted for coffee. Eaten with bread, the bitterness in the leaf vanishes. I always use dandelions as food first.

For medicine, gather the root in the fall. Employed as a diuretic, dandelion has ample potassium to replace what is lost from frequent

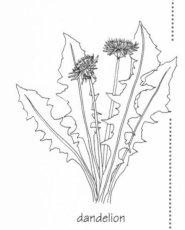

dandelion

urination. Dandelion stimulates liver function, reduces cholesterol, fights diabetes, and stimulates digestion; extracts indicate tumor-fighting capacities on lab-induced breast cancers in mice.

GARLIC *(ALLIUM SATIVUM)*

Even orthodox medicine acknowledges that garlic reduces cholesterol, lowers blood pressure, and decreases the risk of heart attack. But garlic also helps regulate blood sugar levels, is useful in all manner of lung ailments, kills parasites, calms spasms, and relieves inflammation. Did I say it's one of nature's best antibiotic and antiviral agents?

This is the stuff that daily medicine is made of. For greatest benefits, garlic should be eaten *raw*. Unfortunately, some people cannot tolerate raw garlic on an empty stomach. They could try eating it with bread, or taking a garlic footbath. Garlic will retain some of its cardiovascular benefits when cooked, but heat destroys its antibacterial and antiviral qualities. One clove a day is adequate for preventative purposes. Take more for acute ailments such as colds and flus. For external use, always put garlic on a piece of gauze, then lay the gauze next to the skin; otherwise blistering may occur.

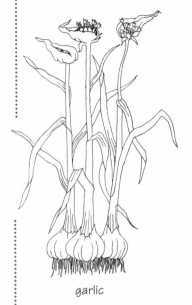

garlic

GINGER *(ZINGIBER OFFICINALE)*

Ginger grows outdoors in the southern United States. The rest of us can grow ginger as a houseplant. It likes ample humidity, good light, and about a month to sprout from a root cutting. A classic remedy for colds, flu, fevers, nausea, menstrual cramps, motion sickness, and hangover, ginger stimulates the circulatory system and acts as a general mild stimulant. To bring heat to a specific area, use a compress of ginger. I use it extensively in food, salves, teas, and baths all through the cold months of autumn, winter, and early spring.

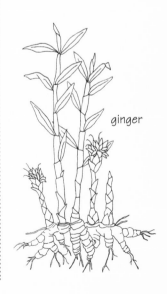

ginger

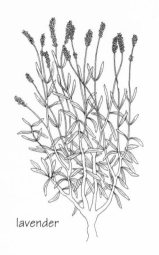

lavender

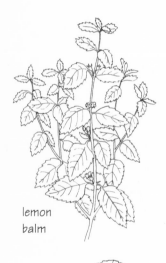

lemon
balm

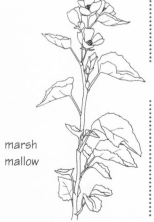

marsh
mallow

LAVENDER (*LAVANDULA ANGUSTIFOLIA* SPP.)

A voluptuous herb, lavender envelops the senses as she heals. Her scent soothes tension, repels insects, and stimulates penile erection. For medicine, gather the flowers when the petals begin to fade. Their uplifting influence calms jittery nerves, relieves headaches, stimulates appetite, and soothes colic. Use the herb freely in baths, compresses, and salves, or in wines, cooking, baking, and beverages.

LEMON BALM (*MELISSA OFFICINALIS*)

Heed this plant's lemony scent: If there's little aroma, there's little medicine. Fresh is best. Lemon balm brings comfort against despair and melancholy. And since illness always brings a measure of sadness, I turn to this herb to heal both spirit and body. Medicinally, the leaves are cooling: They reduce fevers, soothe bruises and aches, heal wounds, calm nervous stomachs, and help heal sores from herpes viruses.

MARSH MALLOW (*ALTHAEA OFFICINALIS* OR *MALVA SYLVESTRIS* SPP.)

Marsh mallow (and to a lesser degree common garden mallow and hollyhocks) soothes irritated mucous membranes throughout the body. It's successful against all manner of digestive disturbances, sore throats, colds, and coughs. It gives a slippery feel to wines and vinegars without altering the taste. The flower petals are a pleasant nibble, but try those little green cheeses where the seeds are made — they are fun!

MULLEIN (*VERBASCUM THAPSUS*)

With mullein, intent is everything: It's used to make magic and to protect from magic. Each part of mullein contains unique medicine. The flowers kill bacteria, and the infused flower oil soothes wounds and earaches.

You can smoke the leaf to open and relax bronchial passages. It is effective against whooping cough, asthma, and bronchitis. Although the whole plant is sedative, the root concentrates this quality. A boiled root tea calms the body inside and out. *Warning:* Mullein seeds are toxic and should never be used for any reason.

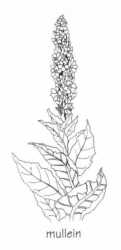

mullein

OATS *(AVENA SATIVA)*

Think of oats as a one-penny moisturizer. Tie a handful of rolled oats in a muslin bag. Moisten the bag and rub it on chapped skin, mild sunburn, eczema, insect bites, and itchy rashes — or toss it into a warm bath. This same soluble gummy fiber soothes the intestinal tract and lowers cholesterol. Eat oat porridge during convalescence to rebuild strength. Both the grain and the oat straw nourish nerve cells and help the body cope with insomnia, anxiety, and nerve disorders such as shingles.

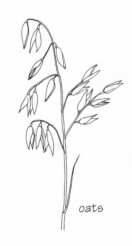

oats

PEPPERMINT, SPEARMINT *(MENTHA X PIPERITA, M. SPICATA SPP.)*

There are many varieties of mints, but peppermint and spearmint are the most popular. I use the milder variety, spearmint, for children. Both are cooling, stimulating, and refreshing in action and flavor. I consider mint a summer herb, as a cup of strong tea will bring on a good sweat and cool the body by evaporation. Slightly antiseptic, mint makes a good mouthwash, wound wash, and sore throat remedy. A simple tea is classic for headache and sinus relief. Ever wonder at the tradition of a complimentary mint at the end of a meal? Mint stimulates digestion and relieves nausea — it helps dispel that overfull feeling and possible indigestion or gas.

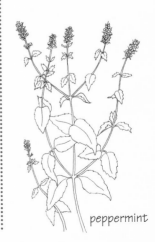

peppermint

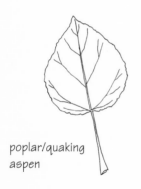

plantain

poplar/quaking
aspen

PLANTAIN (*PLANTAGO MAJOR* SPP., *P. LANCEOLATA* SPP.)

Plantain has followed in mankind's footsteps throughout the world. Perhaps this is a good thing, considering how useful it is. Plantain is a soothing and drawing herb. The leaf is helpful for all manner of external skin irritations and irritations of the digestive system. The seeds are nutritious — they're full of easily assimilated B vitamins. I sprout them throughout the winter months. Used with the husks left on, they are a safe and gentle laxative. The root is an excellent topical dressing to heal stubborn sores. Also known as poor man's spinach, the young leaves may be cut back and lightly steamed. The plant easily grows back from a generous root system, providing you with greens through the summer with no effort other than the harvest.

POPLAR AND/OR QUAKING ASPEN (*POPULUS* SPP.)

Considered a standard remedy in the north woods, this tree grows in dense stands that benefit from being selectively thinned when they are thumb-size saplings. The strongest medicine lies in the inner bark of the trunk. A bitter remedy, poplar contains a substance related to the active ingredient in aspirin (and willow). However, it doesn't irritate the stomach in the same way that refined aspirin will. (**Caution:** As with aspirin, poplar should *not* be taken by children with a high fever.) Poplar buds help break up congestion of the lungs, and aid digestion. They are an old-time remedy for rheumatism, headache, inflamed prostate, and general weakness. A salve made from the sticky buds makes a good deep muscle rub. Make a tincture with the buds of balsam poplar for a natural preservative similar to its commercial counterpart, tincture of benzoin.

RASPBERRY *(RUBUS IDAEUS)*

This is the woman's herb. Drink tea made from the second year's leaf growth to prepare for an easy childbirth and prevent miscarriage. Less astringent and safer for children than its relative the blackberry, raspberry relieves diarrhea and skin irritations. Since the taste of the leaf is somewhat harsh (I like it, though), leaves are seldom used alone, but are the prime ingredient in many herbal formulas. The fruit is a nourishing tonic as well as a gourmet treat. Slightly wilted raspberry leaves may have toxic properties, so be sure to use them fresh or completely dried.

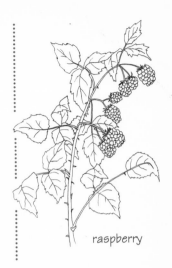

raspberry

CAUTION

Improperly dried leaves of raspberry, strawberry, blackberry, and sweet clovers may contain a compound produced from residual moisture and fungal activity that inhibits blood clotting and may cause internal hemorrhaging. Be sure to use these herb leaves fresh or completely dried only. Some herbalists recommend avoiding them altogether (especially red clover) for several weeks prior to surgical procedures or childbirth.

RED CLOVER *(TRIFOLIUM PRATENSE)*

This was the first plant I let myself "play" with. I tried red clover tea, hair rinse, foot powder, and jelly. I used it for colds and colic, in soups, cakes, cookies, and wine. Finally, I developed a feel for red clover. Don't let the following suggestions limit your "play" with red clover.

Red clover is slightly sweet and cooling. The fresh flowers provide relief from minor inflammations. Internally, red clover rebuilds the body's strength from chronic disorders such as allergies and arthritis. It's been shown to be

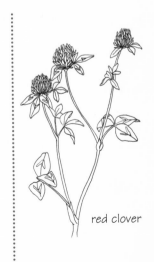

red clover

effective against chemotherapy's side effects. Drunk consistently over a long period of time, it reduces the blood's ability to clot, and while many people have found this herb helps them combat arteriosclerosis, it could prove dangerous during surgery or childbirth. It is wise to remember to take one or two days' rest a week from this herb to help give the body a chance to return to balance, and to avoid it during the last month of pregnancy or before surgery. Gather flowers before they're fully open.

ROSE (*ROSA RUGOSA* SPP.)

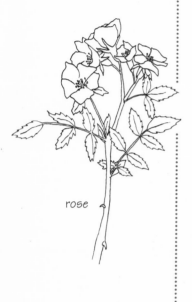

rose

Old-fashioned roses make the best medicines; avoid using hybrid roses. Roses are sweet, astringent, and lightly cooling in medicinal action. Gather the petals, before the flower is pollinated, from the flowers that have a bright sunny yellow center. They have not been pollinated yet and are producing a scent to call to the bees. After pollination, the center anthers turn brown and dry up. The scent is noticeably weaker; soon the petals will fade and drop. Rose petals added to your medicinal preparations will impart a pleasant flavor. To use externally, gather the leaves before the flower buds appear. The petals bring delight to the senses, lighten the spirits, and are mildly astringent. The hips are full of vitamin C, and best gathered after a hard frost. Hidden within the seeds is a storehouse of vitamin E. The whole hips were traditionally set by for late winter to use as a blood purifier.

ST.-JOHN'S-WORT *(HYPERICUM PERFORATUM)*

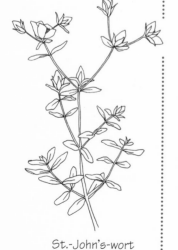

St.-John's-wort

This herb's action is specific to the nervous system. Use it topically to relieve neuralgia or back pain, or to heal cleaned wounds quickly. Drinking the tea calms nervous tension — it can even ease clinical depression — and gives the body an antiviral boost. Look carefully at a leaf and you'll see tiny black dots. This is where the medicine lies. About a week after the flowering, pick a blossom and rub it on your palm. If it leaves red-purple streaks behind, the plant is ready to gather. Gather the top quarter of the whole plant. Some people become sensitive to sunlight after drinking the tea for extended periods of time.

STRAWBERRY (*FRAGARIA VESCA* SPP.)

Strawberry teaches us to pay attention to gathering times. All parts are medicinal, and the medicinal virtue of each part changes throughout the growing season. For example, the unopened blossom is somewhat bitter and astringent, useful against diarrhea and upset stomach. The fully opened flower is fragrant and sweet and stimulates appetite. The stalk in early spring is a tasty nibble; in midsummer it stanches bleeding from a cut. The overall balanced mineral content of strawberry leaf tones the heart and blood vessels. But I'll allow you to discover for yourself when it's best to gather.

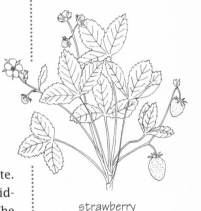

strawberry

THYME (*THYMUS VULGARIS* SPP.)

Modern medicine may have little to offer you against viral infections — but herbalists have thyme. Drink thyme at the onset of a cold or chills to increase the efficiency of the immune system. The tea is also antimicrobial, antifungal, and mildly styptic, making it excellent for external cuts and wounds. Thyme tea warms the stomach, eases cramps, and calms nervous conditions. The plant is so useful that it is known as mother of thyme, or mother's thyme! Avoid frequent large doses of thyme during the first trimester of pregnancy, as it may bring on menses.

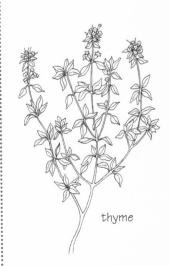

thyme

VIOLET (*VIOLA TRICOLOR, V. ODORATA, AND V. SPP.*)

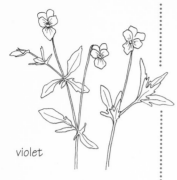

violet

The common Johnny-jump-up and heartsease (purple with heart-shaped leaves) are the two violas most commonly used medicinally. Drying destroys the pleasant aromas and flavors of violet, so use fresh. Syrups will preserve the flower for quite some time, however. Violet syrup will chase a cough away while pampering your taste buds. Fresh violet greens have a peppery taste that lifts otherwise dull salads and dishes. A high-end nutritive plant, violet is a common ingredient in most spring tonics.

WALNUT — BLACK WALNUT OR WHITE WALNUT (BUTTERNUT) (*JUGLANS NIGRA, J. CINEREA*)

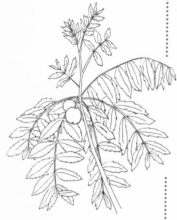

walnut

Working with walnut is an exercise in patience and forethought. The husks, superb against parasites, fungal infection, and skin diseases, will leave your fingers stained brown for months. The nuts contain essential fatty acids, rebuild cellular strength, and are traditionally used to treat eczema internally. They are also notoriously difficult to crack. I use a vise and hammer, or roll over them with my car! Peeling the bark always frustrates me, but the bark is one of the few effective laxatives that is safe to use in pregnancy. Only the leaves are easy to gather, if you can reach them. But no matter: Walnut's reliability in treating these conditions makes it worth the effort. I admit I enjoy meeting the walnut's challenge.

WHITE PINE (*PINUS STROBUS* SPP.)

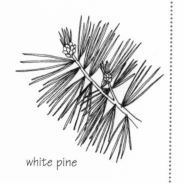

white pine

White pine is a first-aid station wrapped up in a tree. The sap makes an airtight, antiseptic, and pain-relieving bandage. I use it for all manner of burns, scrapes, and wounds. Cover with a tissue to stop the sap from sticking. Fishermen apply warm sap to stubborn splinters to draw them out painlessly. Some people have a skin sensitivity to pine sap — test it on a small patch of healthy skin for possible reaction before applying to a wide area.

The needles are a year-round source of vitamins C and A. They excel at breaking up congestion. Use as tea, steam pot, cough drops, or chest compress. The green bark makes a good splint for sprains, lending both support and pain relief.

Advantages of These Herbs

Obviously, there are many other herbs that can be used. But to start with, the 25 simples discussed in the previous section have several advantages. First, they are common through most of the United States, being easy to grow or readily available commercially. Second, wild populations of these plants are not threatened with overharvesting, as of this writing. Third, all are fairly easy to recognize in the field — with no extremely poisonous look-alikes. And, finally, all have flavors and scents appealing to most beginners.

CHOOSING THE HERB TO USE

The essence of herbal medicine is the quest for balance. Simply put, balance as a chronic state evokes health. Aristotle named it moderation and said "Man must enjoy his moderation, lest that, too, become excessive." At their best, medicinal plants become part of daily living, our food, thus preventing our tendency to swing from one extreme to another.

Seeking Balance

Some plants are balanced, or neutral in themselves, but most plants bring us away from excess because of the balancing work they can do for the body. Generally, I use a plant that has the opposite characteristics of the illness. Between the two (the illness and the herb), balance is found. For example, if the ailment is cold hands, use a plant that generates heat, such as ginger. If the cause of cold hands is poor circulation, look to an herb that promotes healthy circulation, such as strawberry, or to a nutritive herb such as violet to nourish overall health.

As the body moves toward balance, the herbal therapy needs of that body should be reevaluated. Perhaps the symptom of cold hands has disappeared. Is it because winter is over? Because circulation has improved? Each person must heed his own body's signals and rhythms to determine the next step. Perhaps the use of ginger can be discontinued. Perhaps the dose of nutritive herbs can be reduced to a maintenance level, or discontinued for a time to evaluate the results.

No matter what any herbal expert may tell you, you know your body best. Herbal healing is an art. There's no one best way — only the way that works best for the individual. Ultimately, you must find your own balance, or it really is not balance at all.

Working Inside and Out

A common method of herbal therapy is to treat the ailment internally and externally at the same time. To relieve severe colic or gas pain I might have the person rest with a warm poultice of catnip tea on his stomach, as well as drink frequent small sips of catnip tea.

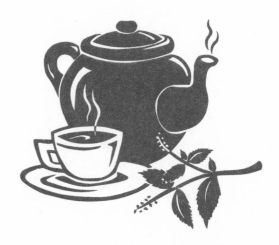

OBSERVE THE FIRST RULE OF FIRST AID

It is a matter of fact that you are assembling your home medicine chest with the hope that you'll never use it — it's your homemade insurance policy. However, the chances are good that you may have to use it, and before you do, be sure to heed the first rule of medicine. Written down by Hippocrates thirty-five hundred years ago, its truth is universally recognized by everyone from ancient ayurvedic Indian practitioners to the modern-day American Medical Association: *First do no harm.*

Assess the Situation Before You Act

Red Cross first-aid training teaches that before you do anything, assess the situation as a whole. Then assess your level of ability to handle it. If it is beyond the scope of your strength, ability, or training, do what you can to stop any imminent dangers that may cause more harm, then go for help. The same holds true at home. Step back and calmly view the situation before embarking on any treatment.

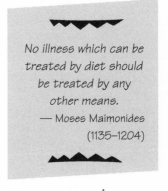

No illness which can be treated by diet should be treated by any other means.
— Moses Maimonides (1135–1204)

Always aim for the lowest level of intervention whenever possible. The body has a remarkable capacity for self-healing — it wants to get better. Your goal should be to aid the body's desire for health, to encourage its own defense mechanisms to kick into high gear. Strive to be noninvasive. Choose rest, fresh air, and water as the first course of treatment whenever possible. The old doctor's prescription for cold relief, "Take two aspirin and plenty of fluids, go to bed, and call me in the morning," is usually just as effective without the aspirin. The aspirin becomes a psychological crutch, so you feel you are at least doing something to fight the illness, and the doctor is doing something to earn his pay. But the water and the rest often do more to stop the cold than the aspirin. Herbs, too, can become a crutch. Use them wisely and sparingly as medicine. Use them freely and liberally as food to build the body's health.

CHAPTER 4
Making Herbal Tinctures

Alcohol is a good preservative for everything but brains.

— Mary Pettibone Poole, *A Glass Eye at the Keyhole*

Tinctures are simple and fun to make. Basically, the process of making a tincture involves extracting the virtues of the plant into an alcohol solution, simultaneously making and preserving the medicine. A mindfully made and stored tincture will generally be potent for about five years. Tinctures are convenient where time constraints or bitter tastes hinder the use of a tea. People often use tinctures for pets, for children, when traveling, or when bedridden.

The money you save from making your own tinctures is almost as good as having a winning lottery ticket. One day, I grabbed my shovel, set my stopwatch, and timed how long it took to make a dandelion root tincture. From digging to clean-up, making 1 quart of tincture took a grand total of 15 minutes of my time. The only cash expense was twelve dollars for the alcohol.

If I was buying that same dandelion root tincture, it would have cost me $4 per ounce on the average — that's $128 per quart! Subtract the $12 spent for the alcohol and I'm still left with a savings of $116 for 15 minutes' work, or $464 per hour!

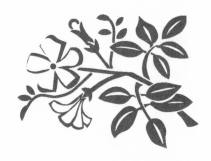

CALCULATING STANDARD DOSE

Tinctures made from the simples recommended in this book are potent medicine. The dose of a tincture is measured in drops. A standard dose many herbalists follow is 1 to 2 drops of tincture for every 5 pounds of body weight, placed in an 8-ounce cup of water. For a baby less than six months old (who's suffering from colic, for example), the mother should take the tincture; the baby will receive the medicine through the mother's milk. For strong-tasting tinctures, disguise the drops in juice or food, or take them sublingually (under the tongue).

Frequency of Use

The frequency and duration of tincture use will vary depending on the illness. For acute conditions such as colds or earaches, take smaller doses more frequently, sometimes as often as ten times a day, with water. For nourishing the overall health or for treating chronic long-term conditions (such as recurring ear infections), take the standard dose two to four times a day for six to eight weeks, or longer if needed.

If an individual is sensitive to alcohol, simply place the drops of tincture into water that is just under the boiling point and let it sit for 5 minutes before drinking. The heat will evaporate most of the alcohol.

HOW TO MAKE A TINCTURE

Making a tincture as described on pages 42–44, with approximately equal amounts of 80-proof alcohol and plant material, yields a product that is roughly 20 percent alcohol. Anything from 15 percent to 25 percent alcohol will store nicely. Use a greater concentration of alcohol and you are not maximizing the herb's potential; use a lesser, and the tincture may mold or turn in storage. Makes about 12 ounces of finished tincture.

Materials

◆ Pint-size glass jar with tight-fitting lid
◆ About 2 cups fresh plant material of your choice
(should fill jar leaving one inch of headroom)
◆ 2 cups 80-proof vodka, brandy, or rum

step 1

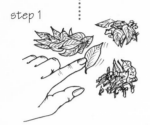

1. Clean and sort through your freshly gathered plants. Discard any yellow, moldy, damaged, or rotten parts. Separate out the parts you will be tincturing — flowers, leaves, or other parts. Wash off muddy roots. You may chop the herbs to help open the cell walls to the alcohol. This speeds up the process, which is useful if you want to start using the tincture in one to two weeks.

step 2

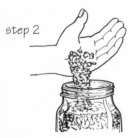

2. Fill the glass jar with the plant material, leaving about 1 inch for headroom.

step 3

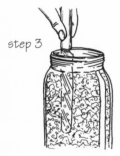

3. Completely cover the herb with vodka, brandy, or rum. Insert a butter knife into the jar and run it around the inside of the jar to release any trapped air bubbles. Add more alcohol to cover. Put on the lid and shake vigorously for about 1 minute.

step 4

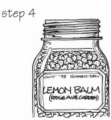

4. Label and date each tincture. If you have room on the label, note what the weather and seasonal conditions were when you gathered the herbs. This will help you identify and track the best gathering times for various herbs (see box).

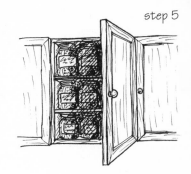

step 5

5. Place the jar in a dark place and let it sit for 3 to 6 weeks. Shake periodically, and check to make sure that the plant material remains covered with alcohol. Add alcohol as needed.

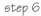

step 6

6. After 3 to 6 weeks have passed and the plant material looks pale, limp, and spent, strain and press the liquid through a piece of cheesecloth into a glass or stainless steel bowl or pitcher, leaving the plant material behind in the jar or on the cheesecloth.

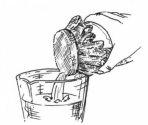

7. Once you've poured out all the liquid, spoon out all the herbs onto the cheesecloth. Wrap the cheesecloth around the herbs, hold over the bowl or pitcher, and wring out any additional tincture.

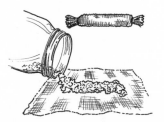

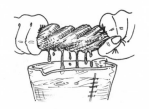

step 7

MAKING HERBAL TINCTURES **43**

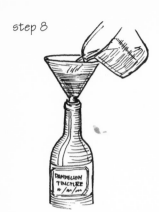

step 8

8. Using a funnel, if desired, pour the tincture into a glass bottle of the appropriate size. Label, date, and store the bottle in a cool dark place.

Now, to be honest, I don't always get to the last three steps right away. I have jars of tinctures several years old sitting on my shelves that still have not been strained. The alcohol keeps the plant preserved. I rather enjoy looking at the preserved plants, and just strain some tincture off to use as needed.

Variations on Method

Using stronger-proof alcohol. If you use 190-proof alcohol to make a tincture, remember you are now working with alcohol that has only 5 percent water. You will have to add some water so the water-soluble components of the herb can be extracted, or use extra amounts of fresh plant material, which contain their own water. The proportion can be increased to one part alcohol to 4 or 5 parts fresh plant material. A simple way to do this is to run the tincture through two or three times.

Thus for a red clover tincture, I'll gather plant material and prepare the tincture once. Two to three weeks later, I'll strain and repack the fluid with yet another picking of red clover. This obviously makes a stronger medicine, so the dosage should be less — roughly 1 to 2 drops per every 10 pounds of body weight. This is a bit more work, but some plants such as ginger, burdock, and poplar buds need the higher concentration of 190-proof alcohol to extract their resins and essential oils.

Juicing the herb. If you happen to have a juicer, you can press the juice from the fresh herb and mix that with an equal amount of 80-proof alcohol to yield a 20 percent alcohol tincture. (One and one-half parts juice to 1 part alcohol will yield a 16 percent alcohol tincture.) Alternatively, you can blend 1 part 190-proof alcohol with 4 parts juice to yield a 19 percent alcohol tincture. (Five parts juice to 1 part alcohol will yield a 15 percent alcohol tincture.)

Using dried herbs. Although fresh plant tinctures are usually preferable, dried plant tinctures are an acceptable alternative. Here are the steps to follow:

1. Grind 4 ounces of the dried herb to a powder using a mortar and pestle.

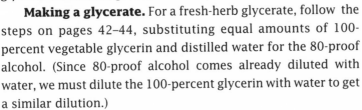

step 1

2. Place the herbs into a 1-pint glass jar.

3. Fill the jar to the top with 80-proof alcohol. Shake vigorously every day. From this point, follow the instructions for fresh herb tinctures (see step 4, page 42), but let the herbs settle before decanting the liquid into the glass jar for storage.

Glycerates Instead of Alcohol

For alcohol-sensitive individuals or for children, consider making a glycerate instead of an alcohol-based tincture. Glycerin is a thick, sweet, and slippery-feeling liquid. It helps mask the taste of bitter herbs such as dandelion, so children like it better. It extracts most plant alkaloids and mucilages (the slippery quality of mallow root), but will not extract resins (found in poplar, white pine, and ginger). Follow the guidelines for the standard tincture dose on page 41, substituting the glycerin for alcohol guidelines.

Making a glycerate. For a fresh-herb glycerate, follow the steps on pages 42–44, substituting equal amounts of 100-percent vegetable glycerin and distilled water for the 80-proof alcohol. (Since 80-proof alcohol comes already diluted with water, we must dilute the 100-percent glycerin with water to get a similar dilution.)

You'll find some herbalists prefer a two-to-one ratio of glycerin to water, since fresh herbs already bring their own natural water to the tincture. So there is some room for experimentation

ONE HERB AT A TIME

Make your tincture only with a single herb at first. Once you have a variety of single-herb tinctures, you can combine them in different proportions as needed. When you find a particularly useful or favorite combination, then consider making the blend from a combination of fresh herbs.

on our part. Do try to keep the final glycerin ratio to at least 25 percent to reduce the risk of spoilage and for safe consumption, since excessive amounts of glycerates may cause diarrhea in sensitive individuals.

To make a glycerate with dried herbs, remember to add extra distilled water to replace the water that has been evaporated out. A proportion of 4 ounces of dried herb, 1½ cups of distilled water, and ½ cup of vegetable glycerin will yield you a 25 percent glycerate. Follow the steps for making dried herb tinctures listed on page 45.

TINCTURE BLEND RECIPES

The following recipes are some of my family's and students' favorites. These represent a variety of blends that are useful to have on hand and ready to use. Once you've tried making some of these, you may want to create your own blends, or adapt these recipes.

Making Blended Tinctures

You will notice that some of these recipes call for gathering flowers in the spring and roots in the fall. Follow the same procedure for making fresh herb tinctures on pages 42–44, only turn it into a two step process: First, tincture your fresh gathered spring flowers and allow the tincture to sit unstrained until you gather your fresh root in the fall. Just remove the spent flowers

---

A NOTE ON MEASURING

The proportions of herbs in these recipes are referred to as parts. How much a part is, is up to you — it could be a gram, an ounce, a pound, depending on how much tincture you want to make and how much plant material you have available. The important thing is that the relative amounts, or parts, are followed closely. It is always more precise to measure by weight, and it's important that you use the same method of measurement for all the ingredients in a particular recipe.

from the tincture, wringing out as much liquid as possible, then use this flower tincture as the base. Now add your roots and begin the tincturing process a second time.

DIGESTIVE BITTERS

This blend stimulates appetite, aids digestion, and reduces nausea. Pregnant women looking to ease morning sickness should leave out the ginger. Instead add a little ginger as a food flavoring. It will still help suppress nausea. Current guidelines state that while ginger is safe for pregnant women when used as a food, it should be used in moderation as a medicine as it may stimulate uterine activity in the early stages of pregnancy. It's also nice for colic, or colds and flus that affect the digestive system. For extreme nausea, take only 1 teaspoon of the standard dose diluted in a cup of water (see page 41), every ten minutes; most of the time this small amount can be kept down. This also makes a nice blend to add to an herbal wine or syrup.

1 part catnip bud or leaf (calms nervous stomach)
1 part grated ginger root (dispels indigestion, flatulence, and nausea)
1 part fall-gathered dandelion root (aids in the absorption of food)
1 part mallow root (soothes the digestive tract)

REJUVENATING FEMALE TONIC

This tonic helps maintain and build the body's strength before and after pregnancy, during nursing, through menopause, and after a miscarriage or abortion; it also eases chronic menstrual cramping.

½ part borage leaf (maintains adrenal health)
½ part lemon balm leaf (lifts spirits)
2 parts fresh raspberry leaf (strengthens female reproductive system)
1 part violet blossom and leaf (tonic to whole system)
1 part burdock root (promotes liver function)
1 part plantain leaf (nourishing and soothing to internal membranes)

COLD SEASON REMEDY

This tastes like medicine — though pleasantly so. I like to take it sweetened with honey and a couple of wedges of fresh lemon. As soon as everyone else around me is getting sick, I start dosing myself with this formula, along with taking a clove or two of garlic. This is the one tincture I always try to have on hand, because when the whole household is sick, I don't always have the time or energy to keep brewing tea.

½ part inner poplar bark (anti-inflammatory and pain relieving)
½ part mullein leaf (helps prevent cold from settling into lungs)
1 part thyme leaf (antiviral and antibiotic)
1 part lemon balm leaf (lifts spirits)
1 part mallow root (soothes inflamed tissues and serves as expectorant)
1 part violet leaf and flower (soothes inflamed tissues and serves as expectorant)
1 part peppermint leaf (reduces nausea and fever, works as stimulant)

DIARRHEA OR DYSENTERY BLEND

This is another good tincture to have on hand ready to use at a moment's notice. Diarrhea can come on quickly and severely and there is danger of dehydration. This formula helps stop the runs and prevent the electrolyte imbalance that can result from severe dehydration.

To administer, take small frequent sips of the standard dose with a tablespoon of vinegar added to it.

2 parts blackberry root (astringent)
1 part alfalfa leaf (helps replace lost minerals)
1 part mallow root (soothes irritated tissues)
1 part red rose petal (astringent)

CHAPTER 5
Making Herbal Oils and Salves

But let us hence, my sovereign, to provide
a salve for any sore that may betide
— William Shakespeare, *Henry III*

Every single day someone in our household reaches for a jar of herb oil or salve. With a family of six, I make herb oils in large batches and store them in the refrigerator so they last as long as possible. With an herb oil in hand, turning it into a salve, ointment, sachet, or balm (all are different terms for essentially the same product) is simply a matter of adding a thickening agent, beeswax being the easiest and most commonly used. Once the word gets out that you make your own oils and salves, expect to make some for friends and relatives. Show them how to use it, and be sure they actually want the product before you give it away: It is heartbreaking to see a jar of your precious home-made salve just sitting on a shelf for years.

HOW TO MAKE AN INFUSED-HERB OIL

When you begin experimenting with this process, I recommend making a basic herb oil with a single herb. Just as with tinctures, most people prefer to make up several different oils and then blend them together when needed to create a blended oil. Sometimes, though, you will have a specific use for an oil or salve in mind and will want to make a blended-herb oil. Following are the steps for making a single-herb oil for external use. The amounts given will make about 5 ounces of herb oil, but you do not need to follow these proportions exactly. How much herb oil you make depends on how much of the herb you have and the desired strength of the finished oil. The basic principle is simply to cover the herbs with oil and allow them to steep.

If you use the preservation techniques I recommend in step 3, the oil should have a shelf life of six months to one year when stored in the refrigerator. Makes about 5 ounces of herb oil.

Materials
- ½ pint widemouthed mason jar with 2-part lid
- About ¾ cup herb of your choice
- ¾ cup oil of your choice
- About 2 tablespoons 190-proof alcohol
- A few drops of balsam poplar tincture (optional) (see pages 42–44)

1. Gather the fresh herbs of your choice. Shake the dirt off the leaves or wash and blot dry the roots. Sort out and discard any diseased plant material. Make a pile of the part of the herb you wish to use. Chop it coarsely until you have about ¾ cup.

step 3

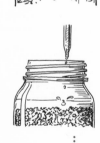

2. Mold and fungus grow easily in oils, so allow the herb to partially wilt overnight to reduce moisture content. The volume of the herb will also reduce.

3. Fill a glass jar with the herbs. Leave about 2 inches of headroom. Cover the herb with oil. Insert a butter knife into the jar and run it along the inside of the jar to eliminate any trapped air bubbles. Make sure the oil covers the herbs completely, you may need to add a little more oil.

I like to float a ½-inch layer of 190-proof alcohol on top (vodka would work also). The alcohol helps prevent airborne molds from turning your oil and helps draw the plant essences into the oil. I also add a couple of drops of balsam poplar tincture on top as a natural preservative. Cover with tight fitting lid and shake vigorously for about a minute. Remove the lid.

4. Cover the jar with four layers of cheesecloth, secure with the outer ring of the jar lid or a rubber band, and place it in a warm dry spot (such as a sunny windowsill or on top of a water heater) for about 2 weeks, or until the oil has taken on the color of the herbs and the alcohol has evaporated. I have also had success setting the herbs in a slow-cooker on a low setting or in a yogurt maker for several days. Some people prefer to simmer their herbs on the stove for a couple of hours. While this does make the oil quickly, I find its end product generally pales in comparison to those of the slower methods.

5. Finally, strain the oil through cheesecloth or a mesh strainer into a bowl, pressing out as much oil from the herbs as possible. Let the oil sit overnight. Decant the oil to separate it from any sediment or water that may have settled to the bottom. To decant, simply pour the top oil off slowly. As the bottom sediment comes to the edge, stop pouring. Let settle. You can use a turkey baster to siphon off the remaining oil resting on top of the sediment. Store the oil in a capped glass jar in the refrigerator or another cool dark place until needed. Label and date the oil.

HOW TO MAKE A SALVE FROM AN HERB OIL

When kept in the refrigerator, salves seem to have a longer shelf life than herb oils — often twice as long, or up to two years.

Materials
- ◆ Double boiler
- ◆ 1 tablespoon (15 ml) beeswax
- ◆ Other nutrients, as desired

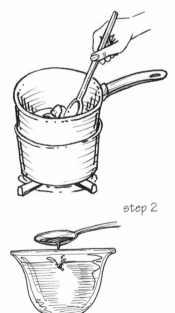

step 1

step 2

1. Gently warm 8 liquid ounces of herb oil in a glass or stainless-steel double boiler. Add 1 tablespoon of beeswax. Experiment with adding small amounts (about ½ teaspoon at a time) of other enriching ingredients, such as lanolin, vitamin E oil, cocoa butter, coconut oil, balsam poplar bud oil, or balsam poplar bud tincture. Add only a few drops of the tincture at a time, or separation may occur.

2. When the ingredients are melted together, check the consistency by placing a drop or two of the salve in ice water. If the salve is thick, it will form into a little ball. If it's thinner, the oil will spread out over the surface. Add small amounts of beeswax (¼ teaspoon at a time) to firm the salve, or slightly larger amounts of herb oil (one teaspoon at a time) to thin the salve.

3. While the mixture is still liquid, pour it into a shallow large-mouthed glass jar, or a container you can easily get your fingers into to reach the salve. Let sit until cool. If salve is not of your desired firmness, place the jar into a hot water bath until the salve is again liquid. Play with adjusting the proportions of oil to beeswax until you are happy with your results. Keep notes; you'll appreciate it for the next batch! Label and date the jar. To store a salve for future use, pour melted beeswax on the top to seal it from decay.

Add a touch of whimsy to your home-made salves by using unusual containers. For example, seashells or a hollowed-out birch log make practical nonreactive containers, and unique gifts.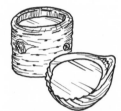

RECIPES FOR OILS AND SALVES

Using these basic techniques, you can make your oils and salves with single herbs or in combinations. If you have a sense of what you will be using the salve for before you start making it, then you can select the most appropriate herbs and proportions for each to treat a particular ailment. Have some fun experimenting to develop your own oil combinations, and discovering your personal favorites. Following are a few of my own favorites.

HOW THICK DO YOU WANT YOUR SALVE?

The consistency, or thickness, of your salve can be varied by the amount of herb oil to beeswax you use. Your choice will depend on how you intend to use the salve. A thicker, waxier salve is best for rubbing into cracks around knuckle joints, or for lip balms and sachets. A softer, oilier salve is preferable for massage oils and liniments, where it will be applied over a larger area of the body.

HUNTER'S HAND AND FOOT RUB

This is a favorite salve for bringing heat to an area and providing a measure of pain relief. Rub on your chest and sinuses to break up congestion, on your feet at the end of a long day, on your hands before going out to work in cold soil, or on sore muscles. It can also be used as a daily application to get rid of those tiny red spider veins that form on legs, arms, neck, and face. *Warning:* Don't use this salve near your eyes or delicate tissues. Use 190-proof alcohol when making this herb oil to be sure to extract the essences of ginger and poplar into the oil.

- 1 part inner poplar bark (reduces inflammation and relieves pain)
- 1 part grated fresh ginger root (increases circulation)

NOT FOR WOMEN ONLY

This blend has a spicy clean scent that appeals to both men and women. Use it as a massage oil or thicken it to make a salve to soothe chapped lips or mild sunburn. My daughter likes to dab a little of the salve behind her ears as a perfume sachet — so does her father, and I like the scent when he does!

- 1 part lavender blossom (spicy scent, topically healing, and antiseptic)
- 1 part wild rose petal (soothing scent, astringent, and anti-inflammatory)

CAUTION ON OILS

Never use essential oils in place of homemade infused oils: They are *not* interchangeable. Essential oils are the concentrated distilled essences of plants; it may take as much as a pound of lavender to make a few drops of essential oil. They are nearly always diluted before use and seldom applied directly onto the skin or used internally. All the recipes for oils in this book incorporate only infused oils. Do not use essential oils in their place unless appropriate reductions in measurements are made and the oils are properly diluted!

ALL-PURPOSE SALVE

This multipurpose salve provides relief to sore muscles, reduces inflammation, heals scrapes, relieves minor burns, and even provides a measure of protection from biting insects. Excellent chest rub to break up congestion.

- 1 part plantain leaf (topically healing and soothing)
- 1 part lavender blossom (antiseptic, topically healing, pain relieving, repels insects)
- 1 part peppermint leaf (cooling, antispasmodic, and pain relieving)
- 1 part thyme leaf (antiseptic and antifungal, increases blood flow to the area, healing and astringent)

GENTLE SALVE

This blend is suitable for all manner of sore or chapped skin that accompanies having babies, including cracked nipples, chapped bottoms, perineal stitches, stretch marks, and diaper rash. It can also be used safely on delicate elderly skin. It relieves inflammation, is mildly antimicrobial, and soothes irritated tissues.

- 2 parts plantain leaf (topically healing)
- 1 part violet flowers (soothing, healing, and antimicrobial in action)
- 1 part mullein flowers (reduces swelling and inflammation)

FAST-HEALING SALVE

This salve promotes rapid cell growth so wounds heal quickly with reduced scarring. Do not use this salve over infected or dirty skin, as new tissue can grow right over the infection, complicating the wound.

- 2 parts St.-John's-wort flower (stimulates nerve endings to heal)
- 1 part balsam poplar buds (antiinflammatory, antiseptic, and paints a thin protective resin over cut to keep wound clean)
- 1 part crushed rose hips (or vitamin E oil: 1 tablespoon vitamin E oil to every 4 tablespoons herb oil)

Optional ingredient: 1 part white pine pitch, for a salve effective against those cracks you get in the sides of your fingers from working in the garden too much (chilblains)

ANTIFUNGAL SALVE

~~~~~

These herbs may be made into a salve, to help heal broken and cracked skin, or a vinegar (see page 66), to help relieve itching when the skin is not broken. Dilute vinegar by two-thirds with water before applying to cracked or open tissues. It stains the skin, as iodine does. This formula works well for athlete's foot, ringworm, and ectopic or eczematous skin conditions.

1   part walnut husks (antifungal)
1   part thyme leaf (antiseptic)
1   part rose leaf (astringent)
1   part plantain leaf (soothing)

BORAGE OIL

~~~~~

The seeds from borage (and evening primrose) contain a special substance called gamma linoleic acid, also known as GLA. GLA (naturally occurring in human breast milk) helps correct metabolic imbalances in the body and inflammations that stem from a degeneration of organic processes. It is most often used to help restore balance during recovery from alcoholism, during weight loss, to ease premenstrual syndrome and arthritis, soothe infantile eczema, and reduce irritable bowel syndrome; it's also a quick remedy for hangovers. Both borage oil and evening primrose oil are readily available at most health food stores — be sure it has been cold expressed and not chemically extracted. The oil should be taken internally several times daily and, for quicker relief, be simultaneously applied externally to the affected regions.

~~~~~

GATHERING MULLEIN

I enjoy picking mullein flowers — it is an exercise in patience that takes me past the work and becomes a form of movement meditation. But if I have a busy schedule which limits the time I can spend picking, then the slow pace becomes frustrating instead of calming. A shortcut is to gather the entire flower spike and chop it up finely. One flower spike is generally enough to fulfill my family's needs for the year. Gather the spike just above the last set of leaves to allow the mullein plant to grow another spike.

▲▲▲▲▲

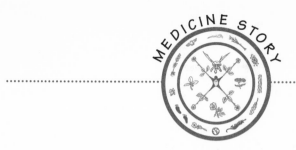

HOW WE GOT MAPLE SYRUP

Once, a beautiful young maiden was taken captive by a warring tribe. She soon realized the journey back to her people was too difficult to manage on her own, so she made up her mind to learn the ways of her captors. Now, her captors were harsh to her at first, but after she learned their language she was no longer treated as a captive, and she was called Moqua.

A young warrior became fond of Moqua and they married. At first, Moqua worked hard to always have a warm fire and good food waiting for her husband when he returned from hunting. But as her skill grew at her tasks she found she could have everything done by midmorning. Then she'd spend the rest of the day visiting with friends. One spring day she was in such a hurry to go visiting, she didn't want to waste time gathering the cooking water.

So instead of getting water to add to the meat pot, Moqua quickly poured the maple sap her husband saved for his evening drink into the pot, thinking, "I'll gather more sap later to replace it — he'll never notice." She put on a big chunk of beechwood so the fire would last a very long time, set the meat pot off to the side to slowly simmer, then left for the rest of the day.

Moqua had such a good time that she didn't notice it was getting dark. She hurried home, worried her husband would be angry that she hadn't replaced the maple sap she'd taken. When she returned, he sat waiting for her, but a grin was on his face. "What did you do to this meat?" he asked. "It is the best I've ever had. Why, I want you to cook it like this every time!"

Puzzled, Moqua peered into the kettle. She saw that the meat was sticky, and it tasted sweet and wonderful. She noticed little grains of something like sand at the bottom and wondered if, perhaps, the maple sap had made this? So she washed her kettle, then poured in the last bit of the maple sap. She set it on the fire to boil. Then she set it outside in the snow to cool. The result was maple sugar. The fame of Moqua's skill in cooking soon spread everywhere. And Moqua's husband always helped her gather and cook the sap every spring to be sure of his wonderful dinners.

Versions of this story are common throughout maple sugar country. Most of this area shares a common linguistic root — the Algonquian. Though each tribe may claim to have been the first to make maple syrup, the ultimate credit goes to Moqua, the captive who made many mistakes.

CHAPTER 6
Making Medicinal Wines and Vinegars

"Just living is not enough," said the butterfly.
"One must have sunshine, freedom, and a little flower."

— Hans Christian Andersen

Winemaking has been around far longer than the specialty homebrewing supply shops that sell all kinds of paraphernalia, from fermentation locks to expensive and delicate yeasts, cadmium tablets, and even glass bottles and corks! Being a tightwad at heart, I wondered just how *did* they used to make wine without all that fancy equipment, and could I replicate the process in my own home?

I headed over to my local library to research an old English and Celtic form of wine called mead. What I found out was that not only were wines once made from fruit, but herbs were added as well, to give unique flavors, scents, and healing properties. I have been hooked on winemaking ever since.

Making wine relies on the slow process of fermentation for preservation. Fermentation happens naturally as plants are left exposed to air and rot. While they do so, airborne yeasts and bacteria break down sugar and starch. Alcohol is excreted in the process. The yeasts and bacteria keep producing alcohol, until eventually the environment becomes toxic to them and they die. This is what forms the sediment in your bottles of homemade wine and vinegar. The trick is to control this process to yield a desirable product.

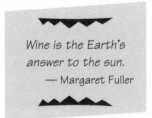

Wine is the Earth's answer to the sun.
— Margaret Fuller

HOW TO MAKE MEDICINAL HERB WINE

It usually takes about 2 months to make a batch of wine from start to finish, but I actually put in only about 2 to 3 hours' effort in all. Fermentation can be smelled by every wild animal living in your county — they also consider wine a delicacy — so find a critter-safe area for your fermenting brew.

When starting out, you will probably want to produce several small experimental batches. Once you have your recipe down, you'll find it is more economical to make larger batches. With experience, you're also likely to want to give the finished wine a longer time to age and mellow. Following are proportions for both small and large batches. Note that the proportions are slightly different for the larger batch.

For small experimental batches:

Yield: about 1 gallon without sediment

1–2	quarts (1–2 liters) fruit (optional)
1½	gallons (6 liters) water
1	pound (400 g) honey (or other sugar source)
1	tablespoon (15 ml) baker's yeast
½–1	pound (200–400 g) herbs
1	pound (400 g) dried fruit

For larger batches:

Yield: About 4 gallons without sediment

4	quarts (4 liters) fruit (optional)
5	gallons (19 liters) water
3	pounds (1 kilogram) honey
1	tablespoon (15 ml) baker's yeast
3–5	pounds (1–2.25 kilograms) herbs
3	pounds (1 kilogram) dried fruit

Equipment:

- ◆ Long-handled stirring spoon
- ◆ Paring knife
- ◆ Masher or grinder, to prepare fruit and herbs (optional)
- ◆ Large crock pot or other container made of glass or stainless steel; or an oak barrel (I've even used a 5-gallon plastic bucket — not my first choice, but better than not making wine at all)
- ◆ Three to four 750 ml bottles for each gallon of wine
- ◆ Containers for siphoning
- ◆ Cheesecloth
- ◆ Rubber bands
- ◆ Plastic tubing

1. Sterilize all the equipment you will use, including the containers for siphoning, with peroxide (see pages 17–18) or by boiling for 10 minutes.

2. Gather your fruits and herbs of choice. Clean them, sorting out and disposing of any debris or moldy- or diseased-looking pieces. Mash or cut the fresh (not the dried) fruit into 1-inch chunks. Cut any herb roots into 1-inch pieces or grind them coarsely. A food processor works well for this.

3. Place all the fruits and herbs into a large ceramic crock or other nonreactive container. (Although many herbalists like to decoct and strain the herbs first, I find that even hard roots such as burdock yield their virtues through fermentation. I simply strain and press out the herbs at the end.) Add the water, honey, and yeast, but make sure your container is only three-fourths full to allow room for expansion. Stir until well dissolved.

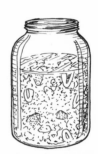

step 3

4. Cover with three layers of cheesecloth to allow the gases to exchange while preventing flies and renegade yeasts from getting in. Secure cheesecloth with a rubber band or string.

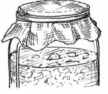

step 4

5. Set in a warm place (about 75°–90°F). Soon you will see bubbles start to rise. This is the start of fermentation, and means everything is working fine. After 5 to 7 days you'll notice the fermentation process noticeably slowing down (the bubbling is less active but not altogether gone).

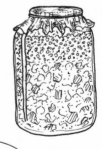

step 5

6. Add the dried fruit. Cover with clean cheesecloth. Let sit undisturbed until all fermentation (bubbling) stops — about 3 to 6 weeks, depending on the temperature.

step 6

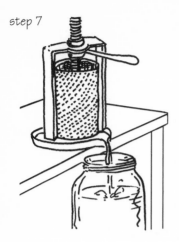

7. Strain all plant material out of the wine, using a press, a rice strainer, or a food mill to extract as much liquid from the plant material as possible. If you do not have any of this equipment, strain the wine through clean cheesecloth, then wrap the herbs in the cheesecloth and wring out the additional liquid; in larger batches, you may get as much as an additional gallon from this squeezing. Let the wine sit undisturbed in the original container or another large nonreactive container covered with clean cheesecloth for 24 hours to settle.

8. You will notice a layer of sediment on the bottom. Either decant the clear liquid slowly and then use a turkey baster to get the last bit out, or set up a simple siphon.

To make a siphon you need two equal-size containers and about 3 feet of ½-inch plastic tubing. Place the container holding the wine on a table, and place the other empty container on the floor. Fill the tube completely with water, pinching both ends to seal it. Hold one end over a sink or extra container at a lower level. Place the other end in the container holding the wine, and then release the tube, allowing the water to flow out until the tube is filled with wine. Then pinch the end of the tube. Transfer that end into the empty container on the floor, and allow gravity to do its work. Monitor the siphon in the wine to make sure it does not get down into the sediment and start siphoning off that as well.

step 8

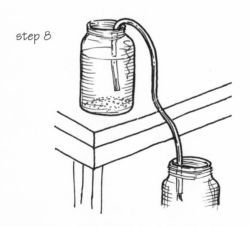

Use a simple siphon to draw the clear liquid from the higher container, leaving the sediment behind.

9. Pour the wine into sterilized wine bottles. I used to cork the bottles right away, but not anymore. If the fermentation isn't fully complete, the gas can pop the cork right out, leaving a big mess to clean up. To ensure complete fermentation, use a small deflated balloon as a test. Simply slip the balloon over the top of the bottle and watch for 24 hours. If there is any fermentation, escaping gas will inflate the balloon. Let the gas out of the balloon, and keep testing until the balloon remains deflated for 24 hours. Then cork, label, and date the bottles. You may cover the cork with melted beeswax to ensure a proper seal.

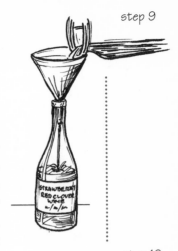

step 9

10. Store your wine in a cool dark place for at least 6 months. This allows for harsh flavors to blend and mellow. Keep corked bottles stored on their sides; otherwise the corks will dry out and there will no longer be a proper seal.

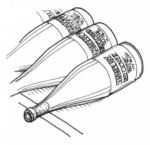

step 10

FAVORITE MEDICINAL WINE RECIPES

Winemaking fosters the creative impulse — have fun mulling over all the possible fruit and herb combinations before making a batch. If you can't decide whether to make lavender-strawberry wine or lavender–rose hip wine, a good way to sample potential flavor combinations is to first make a small pot of tea from the ingredients and do a taste test.

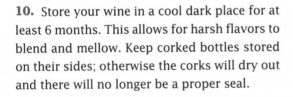

STANDARD DOSAGE FOR MEDICINAL WINE

The standard dose for medicinal wines is 1 to 2 ounces taken one to three times daily as needed. For children, I'll pour just-under-boiling water over the wine and let it rest for 5 minutes before serving. A little sweetener may be necessary.

I like to choose a fruit that has medicinal virtues suitable to the purpose of the wine. For example, for a wine designed to promote cardiac circulation, I would choose to use the circulation-enhancing fruit strawberry instead of raspberry or blackberry.

WINE TONIC FOR IMPROVED CIRCULATION

For fruit:
Fresh ripe strawberries

For herbs, combine:
2 parts red clover blossom (nourishing herb with mild blood-thinning properties)
1 part alfalfa leaf (provides trace minerals)
1 part lavender flower (eases depression and aids digestion)
½ part violet blossom (gentle circulatory stimulant)
½ part whole crushed rose hips (rich source of vitamin E)

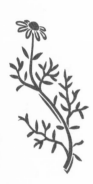

REJUVENATING WINE TONIC

This formula is especially good for rebuilding strength from exhaustion, after pregnancy, from nursing, or after a long illness.

For fruit:
Raspberry, with 1 orange added per 1 gallon water

For herbs, combine:
1 part violet blossom and leaf (nourishing, diuretic, and anti-inflammatory)
2 parts borage leaf (maintains adrenal health)
1 part lemon balm leaf (uplifts spirits)
1 part green oat straw, with developing seed head (nourishes nervous system, soothing)
1 part alfalfa leaf (rejuvenating and nourishing)

GARLIC WINE

Make just enough of this wine for one day's use, since it should be used fresh; many of the active principles in the garlic will be lost by the next day.

  1 fresh clove garlic, crushed
  3 ounces (75 g) wine

Add the crushed garlic to the wine and let it rest for 10 to 15 minutes.

For external use: Apply this wine as a wash, or moisten a cloth and lay the garlic wine on as a dressing.
For internal use: Sip the 3-ounce glass of wine slowly throughout the day.

THE ORIGINS OF GARLIC WINE

The use of garlic wine dates back to the Greek physician Dioscorides, who administered it to the Roman Army. Dioscorides was also a famous Greek herbalist, responsible for devising the method of cataloging medicinal items still used by modern pharmacists.

His list of recommended applications for garlic wine is impressive: treating chronic coughs, healing wounds cleanly, preventing infections, dispelling toxic poisoning from bites of bees and scorpions, preventing and eliminating internal parasites, preventing food poisoning, clearing the arteries, preventing the spread of infectious diseases, and as a disinfectant wash. Garlic poultices were used for treating wartime injuries all the way up through World War I, when it was applied as a wound dressing, saving the limbs and lives of tens of thousands of soldiers.

Digestive Bitters

Bitters help balance overly sweet and salty diets. They activate digestive enzymes and bring warmth to the digestive process, helping the body break down and properly absorb the nutrients in our food. Most often they are used moderately in cooking or drunk just before eating.

BITTERS 1

For fruit:

Apples, or an equal amount of apples and oranges (quartered)

For herbs, combine:

1 part fall-gathered dandelion root (promotes secretion of bile and helps with digestive absorption)

1 part mallow root (soothing)

1 part burdock root (aids liver function)

½ part thyme leaf (stimulates digestion)

½ lavender blossom (stimulates digestion)

½ part gingerroot — if you like a ginger "bite" and want a bitters that is aggressively warming (perhaps to balance a vegan diet), double the amount

BITTERS 2: DANDELION WINE

Dandelion wine makes an excellent digestive bitters all on its own. Take a 1-ounce serving of the wine fifteen to twenty minutes before eating. It can also be taken after a heavy meal to aid digestion.

For fruit:

1 lemon and 1 orange per 1 gallon (4 liters) of water

For herbs:

Dandelion flowers, picked early in the day

BITTERS 3

For children or those with sensitive, spasmodic stomachs.

For fruit:

Apples

For herbs, combine:

1 part catnip flower (calms nervous stomachs)

1 part dandelion flower (aids digestive process)

1 part mallow root (soothes irritated tissues)

1 part plantain leaf (soothes and heals)

Flower Wines

Basically any edible flower can be made into a wine. Some flowers are slightly insipid; adding a lemon will give their wines a little lift. You can also add a few walnut leaves for a drier, higher-tannin wine. One popular flower wine is, of course, rose petal, but lavender flower is equally sublime. A favorite of mine is blue wine made from borage, violet, and lavender flowers, with a couple of handfuls of crushed almonds thrown in for flavor. The wine will have the medicinal attributes of the flowers you choose.

CAUTION

Red clover leaf and blossom, along with other herbs that contain coumarin glycosides, including strawberry, blackberry, and raspberry leaves, may form a toxic dicoumarol molecule when improperly dried. Dicoumarol reduces the blood's ability to clot. Pharmaceutical medicine uses it as a powerful anticoagulant. To avoid a potentially serious situation, always be sure to use only fresh or thoroughly dried and properly stored herbs for your wine- or vinegar-making process.

The leaves and seeds of apples, apricots, plums, cherries, and peaches contain a natural form of cyanide, hydrocyanic acid, which is released as that plant part is broken down. Do not add these leaves or seeds to your wine.

MEDICINAL VINEGARS

On the day my daughter was due to be born, I thought I'd get ahead and make a big batch of strawberry wine before things got crazy with a new baby. I gathered strawberries that morning, and by lunchtime I had a 10-gallon crock filled and fermenting. Just when I thought I could sit back and relax, labor started.

Later that day an 8½-pound baby girl was born! She was perfect in every way, and as babies will, she kept us hopping. But the wine turned out to be far from perfect.

In my haste to make the wine, I hadn't sorted out the blemished strawberries, since they had all just been freshly gathered. Then I let the wine sit for several weeks before I finally got around to looking at it. When I took off the cheesecloth, the rapidly fermenting brew had turned to vinegar. My first thought was to throw it all away; it certainly wasn't useful as wine. But curiosity got the best of me and I let the brew finish fermenting. I strained it and decanted off the sediment, and ended up with a five-year supply of the best strawberry vinegar this side of the Mississippi.

It turns out that wine *wants* to sour. This is part of the natural fermentation process. If you add fruit that is not sound, chances are good that bacteria are already present on it. I like making vinegar because I can use up otherwise discarded bruised peaches, apple peelings, and herb stems, thus extending the yield from my harvest.

How to Make Medicinal Vinegars

Since producing my first unplanned batch of vinegar, I've found a few techniques to help ensure a good medicinal vinegar. Following is a recipe to ensure a good batch of vinegar.

Yield: About 2 gallons without sediment
- 2 gallons (8 liters) water
- 1–1½ pounds (400 to 600 g) of herbs
- 2–3 quarts (2–3 liters) fruit
- 1 tablespoon (15 ml) baker's yeast
- ½ cup (125 ml) mother vinegar (see page 14)
- 1 pound (400 g) honey (or other sugar source)

1. Sterilize all the equipment you will use with peroxide (see pages 17–18) or by boiling for ten minutes.

2. Gather your fruits and herbs of choice. Sort and discard any black or obviously molded parts on the fruit. A little bruising or discoloration (brown apple peelings) is okay, however.

3. Since the process of "souring" happens fairly quickly, take one gallon of the water and use it to brew the herbs into a strong tea. Strain and press out excess tea from the plant material. Ultimately this makes a stronger medicinal vinegar than if you first make the vinegar, then add the herbs to vinegar as you would with a tincture. Also, since the herbs are part of the vinegaring process, the resulting acid content is higher, decreasing the chance of spoilage. Add in the other gallon of water, and let cool to room temperature.

4. In a 3-gallon crock or other nonreactive container, combine the 2 gallons of room temperature herb tea, fruit, yeast, mother vinegar, and honey.

5. Cover with three or four thicknesses of clean cheesecloth secured with a rubber band or string. Store in a warm place between 75° and 90°F.

6. A key to vinegar is exposure to air. Remove the cheesecloth and skim off any surface scum that may develop. Then give the brew a good stir (use a nonreactive spoon) once or twice every day for about one week. Skim off any froth that rises from the stirring. Replace the cheesecloth cover when done stirring and skimming.

7. When the fermentation is finished, the bubbling will stop and the brew will no longer be frothy. It will smell and taste sour. This takes about one week. Strain out the fruit. Let settle overnight, covered with the cheesecloth. Remove the cover and slowly pour off the clear liquid from the bottom sediment. Use a turkey baster to carefully get the last bit of clear vinegar out, or set up a simple siphon (see page 60). The bottom sediment may be saved to act as the mother vinegar in your next batch of vinegar.

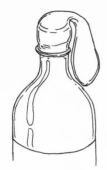

8. Pour the vinegar into the bottles. Slip a small deflated balloon on top to monitor for possible fermentation. When the balloon remains deflated for 24 hours, fermentation has stopped. Now you may safely cork the bottles. Cover the cork with melted beeswax to ensure a proper seal. Label and date your bottles. Store the bottles on their sides.

9. You can use the vinegar right away, but just like wine, the flavors of herb vinegars mellow and blend upon aging. Try to wait at least three months before using, if possible.

Guidelines for Use

Medicinal vinegars can be used in the same ways that the comparable herb wine or tincture would be used. They are excellent for people who are intolerant to alcohol. A tablespoon of honey and a tablespoon of herb vinegar in a cup of water makes a refreshing beverage — hot or cold — to help normalize digestion, restore the acid-alkali balance, and provide energy. They may be freely used internally and externally.

Herbal vinegars are generally not as medicinally potent as their alcohol counterparts, but when made with herbs that nourish the organs such as alfalfa, violet, or red clover, herbal vinegars make a tonic superior to a comparable alcohol tincture. Tonics are a cornerstone to slowly build and maintain a healthy condition. They counteract nutrient deficiency, rebuild vitality, and should be mild and nourishing. Tonics are best taken daily and regularly. Herbal vinegars make a tasty addition to a diet, and their mild nature allows them to be used as a tonic. In fact, I keep taste foremost in mind when putting a vinegar brew together. Lavender, borage, violet, and rose all make sublime vinegars; the more culinary herbs such as ginger and thyme are great, as well.

It is difficult to determine the percentage of acid for homemade vinegars. Commercial vinegar is always 5 to 7 percent, and is strong enough to use as a preservative for pickling. Never use homemade vinegar to pickle vegetables or fresh herbs. The water content of the fresh plants may be just enough to tip the scale too far away from the acid content necessary to preserve the vinegar and prevent botulism from growing. Should you be concerned about a low level of acid, try adding a touch or two of 80-proof alcohol to enhance the preservation.

Although I have often read that medicinal vinegars don't last much longer than six months to a year in storage, I've not found that to be true of well-made homebrewed vinegars. A friend of mine recently used a ten-year-old bottle of homebrewed blackberry vinegar against an intestinal flu that had upset her whole family. She found it very viable indeed.

HIGH-CALCIUM BREW

Vinegar is an excellent medium for carrying calcium into a formula. To make a high-calcium vinegar, incorporate herbs high in this nutrient such as alfalfa, fresh raspberry leaf, and red clover. Another good source is crushed and dried eggshells. Calcium will naturally leach into the vinegar solution until it reaches the saturation point.

CHAPTER 7
Making Syrups and Lozenges

But they whom truth and wisdom lead
Can gather honey from a weed.

— William Cowper, *Pine-Apple and Bee*, 1779

In my opinion, jams and jellies cry out for a little herbal lift. Plain old strawberry rhubarb jelly is fine, but what if you added a touch of mint? or lavender? Yummm! What if you made a lavender syrup to use as a medicine? Wouldn't that be yummy, too? Perhaps it is simply my sweet tooth speaking, but I get immense satisfaction from sharing my homemade violet syrup on top of a big stack of cattail pollen pancakes with friends. It is the best way I know of to turn another person on to the delights of herbalism. And I can make my family's medicine so tasty that it is easily disguised as food. Thus our food becomes our medicine.

MAKING MEDICINE PLEASANT TASTING

Syrups disguise the bitter or strong taste of herbs such as dandelion, white pine, raw garlic, and poplar bark. When a syrup is administered straight from the spoon, children don't notice the bitter until after they swallow the medicine. And somehow, the residual sweetness left in the mouth compensates for the bitter taste — enough so that my children, at least, always ask for another spoonful. Try medicinal syrups for anyone who simply cannot or will not tolerate a bitter or strong flavor. Syrups excel at soothing sore throats, coughs, most digestive upsets, and sudden fatigue. However, the high sugar content makes them a poor choice for treating chronic fatigue, nutritive imbalances, or deep-seated chronic disorders such as diabetes.

HOW TO MAKE A SIMPLE MEDICINAL SYRUP

I'll share with you a process that is by far the easiest way to turn any plain syrup into an epicurean feast. It's good for you, too.

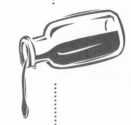

> 1 cup (225 g) water
> ½ ounce (about 2 cups) (250 ml) fresh herb leaf or flower, or
> ½ ounce (about ½ cup) (50 ml) herb root or bark (reduce by half if using dried herbs)
> 1 cup (250 ml) honey, maple syrup, rice syrup, or other sweet syrup

1. Bring water to a boil.

2. Remove from heat and add herb leaf or flower. (If you are using root or bark, do not remove from heat, but allow to simmer over low heat until water is reduced by one-half.)

3. Let stand for about 30 minutes.

4. Strain out herbs, reserving liquid in a saucepan. You now have a very strong cup of tea.

5. Add honey or other syrup to the reserved liquid. Simmer over very low heat on the stove or in an electric warmer that maintains a temperature between 90° and 100°F until most of the liquid is evaporated and the liquid is close in consistency to what the syrup was originally.

6. Bottle, label, and store in a cool dark place or the refrigerator.

FASTER THAN COFFEE

Try starting your day with a cup of instant zing. To make this concoction, add 1 tablespoon of homemade ginger-maple syrup to a cup of hot water. Add a squeeze of lemon. This delicious blend will help kick-start your day without leaving any caffeine jitters to follow.

An Even Simpler Syrup!

Here's a even simpler method for making syrup, using fruit jelly as the sweet base.

1. Make ½ cup (125 ml) of a strong herb tea.

2. Mix tea well with one cup of fruit jelly of your choice. Apple jelly allows the flavor of the herbs to come through the most. Allow it to stand overnight in your refrigerator before using.

This is a good method to use if you're testing a new herb combination and are uncertain about the flavor. I often try out my experiments this way before using them in a more complicated recipe.

You can also make a simple herb jelly by adding ½ cup of fresh, finely chopped herbs and flowers to a fruit jelly. Let stand overnight to give the flavors a chance to blend.

HOW TO MAKE SUGAR-FREE SYRUPS

Low methoxyl-type pectin powders are derived from citrus peels and pulp. They can be used to make jams, jellies, and syrups that rely on calcium to bind and gel rather than sugar (like regular pectin jellies). You can usually find this type of pectin in health food stores: Pomona and Universal are two brand names to look for. When you open the box you'll find two packets, one with pectin, one with calcium. The calcium must be dissolved in water; a small amount of this mix is then added to the recipe.

Selecting Suitable Herbs

To make a syrup using a low methoxyl-type pectin, it's best to use fresh and uncooked herbs. Fresh herbs help give a creamy texture to the recipe, while dried herbs merely seem gritty in comparison. Since the syrup is basically uncooked, delicate flower and herb essences are preserved, plus heat-sensitive vitamins like A and C will not be destroyed. For long-term keeping, however, you will have to store the finished product in the freezer. Try this recipe with all manner of herbs and flowers: peppermint, rose, red clover blossom, lavender, lemon balm, violet — any pleasant-tasting herb or flower. You can even use hard fruits such as rose hips if you cut the blossom ends off the hips first, then whir the hips in the blender with water until you get a milkshake consistency. Let stand for about 2 hours, then strain out the seeds through a sieve. Use this strained liquid to make your syrup. And of course there are all kinds of delicious fruits you can add to give an extra dimension to the flavor of the herbs. Try a lavender and orange juice concentrate blend or apple mint jelly to stimulate digestion. Rose petal, lemon balm, and strawberry is a centering, calming blend. Sweet cherry and lemon thyme syrup is sure to soothe a sore throat and ease coughs. Keep in mind how you will use the syrup as you create your recipes.

> 2 cups (500 ml) of fresh herb or herb-fruit combination
>
> Lemon juice to taste (add ½ teaspoon [2.5 ml] at a time)
>
> 1 cup (250 ml) water
>
> 1 teaspoon (5 ml) methoxyl-type pectin powder

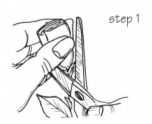

step 1

1. Prepare 2 cups of herb or herb-fruit combination. Flower petals like rose or dandelion are bitter at the base. When you gather them, pull the petals up in one hand and clip off the base with a pair of scissors held in the other. This takes about 15 minutes — the same time allotted for the normal coffee break — and is infinitely more relaxing.

2. If you wish to add lemon juice, combine it with the fresh herb or petals in a blender. Blend well. It may be necessary to add a little water to get the desired consistency, which should be like a milkshake. Remove from blender and set aside.

3. Bring water to a boil. Put it in the blender and add pectin powder. Blend 1 to 2 minutes, until all powder is dissolved.

4. Add the blended herb mixture to the hot pectin mixture in the blender and process on low for 1 minute.

5. You do not need to add any sugar, but if you want to add sweetener for your own personal taste, add now and blend on low until just mixed.

6. Add ½ teaspoon calcium water (from envelope in pectin mix). Blend again just enough to mix well.

7. Fill three 1-cup freezer-safe containers about two-thirds full and let stand at room temperature for 1 to 2 hours. Store in the refrigerator. This syrup will keep for about three weeks. If, when you go to use it, you discover that it has jelled too much, reheat it and add more water and herb (tea). If it hasn't jelled enough, reheat and add a little more pectin.

To save the syrup longer, so you can open up a jar of this summer sunshine during a January blizzard, store it in the freezer and let it thaw about an hour before serving.

To make jam. By adding a little extra pectin to this recipe, you'll end up with a wonderful no-cook freezer jam.

HOW TO MAKE PASTILLES AND LOZENGES

Pastilles are made with plant powders combined with sugar and a binding agent. Pastilles are dried rather than cooked so the plants retain delicate essential oils. They come in handy for relieving sore throats and mouth sores, or for coating and soothing the stomach for long periods of time. I truly felt that I was free of the tyranny of over-the-counter medicines when I made my first batch of homemade cough drops.

Human names for natural things are superfluous. Nature herself does not name them. The important thing is to know this flower, look at its color until the blueness of it becomes as real as a keynote of music.
— Sally Carrigher, Home to the Wilderness (1973)

Pastilles

This is a great project to do with children. Just put down a protective cloth on and under the table to help with cleanup, then have fun with your herbal play dough.

½ cup dried herbs of your choice (try violet or
rose petal to soothe a sore throat, mint leaf
or lavender blossom to ease upset stomachs,
plantain leaf for stubborn mouth sores)
Maple syrup or honey

1. Pulverize your dried herbs in a mortar, then strain them through a sieve to get a fine powder.

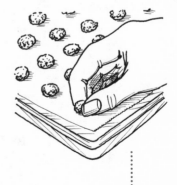

2. Mix the powder with just enough maple syrup or honey to form a ball. It helps to add a mucilaginous plant such as dried marsh mallow root or gum tragacanth (available at many health food stores) to act as a glue. To firm up the consistency, add in more powdered herb ½ teaspoon at a time. Powdered sugar will also absorb excess moisture and sweeten the mixture, and could be added, also ½ teaspoon at a time. Consider adding a pinch of finely chopped balsam poplar buds. The resin helps bind the pastilles, soothe sore throats, and break up congestion, though its flavor is strong.

3. When the mixture is firm enough to hold its own shape, mold into small ¼-inch balls. Use right away, or place on a sheet of waxed paper on a cookie sheet and let sit for 12 to 48 hours to harden. Once hard, the pastilles will last longer in the mouth. Wrap each pastille individually to save for future use. Store in a cool dry place.

Lozenges

Making your own cough drops similar to the ones you can buy in the store is easy. It's basically like making an herbal candy.

> 1 ounce (25 g) dried herb, such as thyme, poplar bud, or ginger
> 1½ cups (375 ml) water
> 2 pounds (800 g) refined sugar

1. Combine herbs and water in a saucepan and simmer steadily over low heat for about 10 minutes. Strain liquid into another pan.

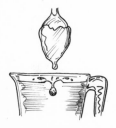

2. Add the sugar to the liquid and bring to a boil. Allow to boil until the mixture reaches 265° to 270°F on a candy thermometer and a few drops form a hard ball when dropped from a spoon into cold water.

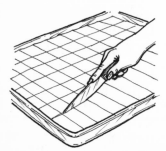

3. Pour mixture into a well-greased 10" x 14" oblong glass or stainless steel cake pan. As soon as it is cool enough to hold its shape, cut it into square lozenges. Wrap each lozenge individually in waxed paper and store in a cool dry place until needed.

Variation. To make a lozenge with a tincture, substitute 1 liquid ounce of the tincture for the dried herb, and reduce the amount of water to ¾ cup. The high temperature will destroy volatile oils such as those found in lemon balm and peppermint. The best way to use a tincture is to simply add it as soon as the sugar mixture is removed from the heat and before it is poured into the pan. When I tried to make a pine sap cough drop, the sap separated out from the sugar, and the method did not work at all. Still, it's worth experimenting with.

CHAPTER 8

Symptoms and Remedies:
An A–Z Guide

▼▼▼▼

Ad sanitatem gradus est novisse morbum.
(When the illness is known, it is half cured.)

— Latin proverb

Now that you know the healing capacity of the herb and how to prepare it for use, you are halfway to being ready to use that herb for a home remedy. Before you begin, however, take the time to understand the characteristics of the illness or condition. The best herbal remedy in the world is no help when used inappropriately. The following general guidelines will help you learn how to use your herbal remedies safely and effectively. Neither the list of ailments nor the guidelines are fully comprehensive. There are many other complaints herbs can be used for; these only represent some of those easiest treated at home. You'll notice that I include several different choices of remedies using the 25 herbs discussed in this book. When possible, try the gentler course of treatment first; fresh air, water, good food, and rest. Select the remedy that has the most relevant action, and that you have available.

Remember that herbal remedies should not be used as a substitute for consultation or treatment by a duly licensed health care professional. When in doubt, seek advice, especially if you are currently taking a pharmaceutical prescription. Many physicians realize that an increasing number of patients are using herbs, and they will at the very least appreciate your being up front about what you are taking. Many can advise about possible herb-drug interactions, and some may even support your efforts to take an active role in your health.

ALLERGIES (HAY FEVER)

Over-the-counter allergy medicine is one of the pharmaceutical industry's best moneymakers. These medications excel at suppressing symptoms, but do little to help the body build a balanced defense system. In fact, they can start a vicious cycle of dependency, ultimately pushing you into seeking even more expensive prescription treatment.

Herbal treatment of allergies involves a three-step process:

1. Avoid exposure. Try to avoid exposure to the allergen whenever possible.

2. Build your natural defenses. Work to build a balanced defense system by using daily doses of fresh, mineral-rich herbs before the allergies manifest themselves. People have found relief from an entire hay fever season by eating abundant amounts of violet greens, dandelion greens and root, along with burdock root in the early spring. These herbs also help the liver break the allergens down into harmless compounds. Keep the regimen up as the season progresses with fresh alfalfa, plantain greens, red clover, and rose hips.

Another old-time remedy is to eat comb honey in four-day cycles several weeks before the hay fever season begins. Local comb honey is considered best. This has varying results, but is so pleasant that it is certainly worth a try.

3. Ease the symptoms. Use steam pots for inflamed stuffy sinuses. Put a handful of decongestant herbs such as mullein, peppermint, and white pine needles into a pot of boiling water. Remove from the heat, drape a towel over your head and the pot, then breathe deeply for several minutes. Take the herb water from

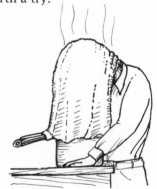

HERBAL ANTIBIOTIC PREPARATIONS

♦ **Garlic-infused wine.** Chop garlic, cover with wine, and let rest for several hours.

♦ **Garlic honey.** Prepare as above, substituting honey for wine. Excellent for cold sores.

♦ **Garlic lemonade.** Prepare as above, substituting honey lemonade for wine, to make a refreshing beverage.

♦ **Garlic water.** Crush 2 large cloves in a quart of water. Let sit for about 6 hours. This may be used on sensitive areas, and internally as a douche.

the steam pot and use it as a nasal spray if you are working or traveling.

Bathe sore, irritated eyes with an infusion of plantain leaf, or bruise the fresh leaves and place them directly on the eyelids for several minutes.

ANTIBIOTICS (herbs to use during and after a course of treatment)

Antibiotics are overprescribed in this country. This is partly the fault of the patient who demands them, and partly the fault of the current medical system that allots only fifteen minutes for a doctor's visit, which leaves little time for patient education. Though the decision to prescribe antibiotics rests with the physician, the responsibility to take them rests with the patient. There are few practices as harmful to your health as taking an antibiotic treatment only until the symptoms disappear — always finish the course of treatment once started.

I heartily recommend you question your doctor if he prescribes antibiotics. Remember the doctor is giving advice, not a law set in stone, and assumes you know nothing. I ask the physician to rate the seriousness of the problem on a scale of one to ten. That helps me understand the situation. I also make it clear that I would prefer to use rest and simple therapies first. Once doctors understand that I am willing to take an active role in healing, I find most will go so far as to offer advice on how to work with alternative treatments — as long as they feel the ailment is not life-threatening.

When a physician gave my three-month-old son's earache a five on the scale, he helped me decide to treat the earache with home remedies first, and to use antibiotics only if the condition worsened. However, when I developed an abscess while nursing and in just a few hours found the whole breast red and inflamed, while my temperature spiked quickly up to 103°F, I was relieved to have the option of antibiotics available.

Replenish healthy bacteria. Antibiotics act indiscriminately in the body, killing off both harmful and beneficial bacteria. Our body relies on certain helpful bacteria to aid digestion and keep other harmful bacteria at bay. To keep a constant replenishment of healthy bacteria in your body, eat at least one 8-ounce serving of plain yogurt every day during and for about

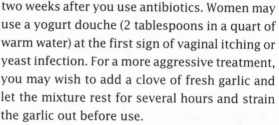

two weeks after you use antibiotics. Women may use a yogurt douche (2 tablespoons in a quart of warm water) at the first sign of vaginal itching or yeast infection. For a more aggressive treatment, you may wish to add a clove of fresh garlic and let the mixture rest for several hours and strain the garlic out before use.

Herbs to aid digestion. Antibiotics disturb digestion. Drink teas that soothe and aid the process such as mallows, plantain, and catnip; or combine ginger, peppermint, thyme, or lavender with mallow root. Sweeten freely with honey.

Herbs to rebuild strength and immunity. After a course of antibiotics is finished, help rebuild your body's immune system with herbs that enhance its functioning. Especially beneficial are raw garlic and thyme, taken in six-day cycles (allow one day of rest from treatment).

The combination of illness and antibiotic leaves your body depleted of nutrients and vitality. Rebuild your strength quickly with dandelion and violet salads or soups, morning oatmeal, alfalfa or plantain seeds or sprouts sprinkled on your food, young plantain leaves lightly sautéed in walnut oil, or cups of nourishing herb teas such as oat straw, borage, red clover, strawberry leaf, and alfalfa.

ANTISEPTICS

Nature generously provided us with thousands of plants with antiseptic value. Antiseptic action from a whole plant is generally milder than that from the plant's essential oil, and so is better to use for minor conditions or as a preventative. For quicker, more immediate action, the essential oil may be used (usually in a diluted form). I strongly suggest you reference a book on essential oils before use, as they are extremely potent substances.

Burdock. Decoct the roots and/or seeds for a skin wash that is unparalleled in its ability to heal chronic skin disorders such as boils, cysts, open ulcers, and scaling eczema. Lay the herb on as a poultice and wrap with a warm towel for such stubborn-healing sores.

Garlic. Nature's broad-spectrum antibiotic, antifungal, antiparasitic, antiprotozoan, and antiviral agent. Research shows that raw garlic extracts act more effectively in rats than the common antibiotic tetracycline! Garlic owes its incredible powers to a compound called *allicin,* which is tricky stuff. You have to chop into it to release its action. Also, the allicin is highly unstable; left alone, half of it will degrade within three hours at room temperature, and it will all nearly vanish within twenty-four hours. Heat completely breaks down allicin within twenty minutes. Forget about using garlic capsules — their allicin component is negligible (although they do contain compounds effective in lowering cholesterol).

Honey. For a quick dressing, smear the affected area with pure honey. Honey is a powerful antibiotic in its own right. Avoid applying straight honey on dry, chapped, or flaky skin, as it may worsen the condition.

Lavender. A useful wound herb, lavender's name comes from the Latin *lavare,* "to wash." Lavender tea is excellent for all manner of external skin ailments, as a mouthwash, and in an ointment for mild burns, cuts, and scrapes.

Poplar bark. Though its antiseptic action is comparatively mild, poplar combines anti-inflammatory action and pain relief for a triple-power-packed punch. Poplar works best in herbal combinations such as poplar-plantain to heal bruises quickly, poplar-marsh mallow for gastric inflammations, and poplar-garlic for inflamed bug bites and scrapes.

Thyme. Thyme is a favorite internal remedy for infections and inflammations. Its active compound, thymol, is exceptionally antiseptic. Add fresh thyme to soups and stews during illness, as well as drinking the medicinal tea. Thyme tea makes an excellent gargle for strep throats, and can also be added to the bath and used in compresses and footbaths.

White pine sap. Apply the sticky sap right onto cuts, scrapes, burns, and wounds for instant pain relief, antiseptic action, and a bandage. Excellent to use in the field, especially over large scrapes. No white pine tree handy? I have found that the extruded resins from white and black spruce; red, jack, pitch, and yellow pines; tamarack; and the north woods favorite, balsam fir, to be just as effective.

Other herbs. Those that demonstrate antiseptic activity include ginger root, lemon balm leaf, mullein leaf and flower, peppermint leaf, rose petal, St.-John's-wort leaf and flower, violet leaf, and walnut leaf.

APHRODISIACS

Lavender. Massage your partner with a lavender massage oil. Lavender has traditionally been considered a sensual herb; simply inhaling its essential oil has been shown to excite penile erection and maintain it for longer periods of time.

Rose. This flower has always been associated with love. Its subtle action lies in the essential oil of the flowers; a simple bouquet of rose and lemon balm leaves placed in a room will help dispel nervous anxiety and gladden the heart. Sipping rose petal wine also stirs the heart, but be careful, for — as they say — alcohol increases the desire while stealing the ability.

Thyme. European tradition called for young men to drink thyme tea before they were wed to increase their sexual interest — which was, perhaps, more important in the days of arranged marriages. I know several men who wholeheartedly believe that this formula works and imbibe thyme tea (or thyme honey) freely and regularly, to their satisfaction.

Other herbs. In traditional Chinese medicine, burdock root has a reputation for increasing sexual desire; in the Middle East, alfalfa was said to make both man and horse virile.

ASTRINGENTS

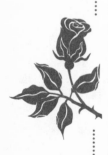

Use an astringent wash to tighten the skin and mucous membranes, and to check excessive body secretions. They are useful for checking bleeding, tightening and relieving hemorrhoids, and treating swollen tonsils, varicose veins, and diarrhea.

Many astringents are high in tannin, the substance that makes your cup of black tea leave a dry aftertaste in the mouth. Rose leaf, poplar bark, raspberry leaf, and blackberry leaf are strong astringents. Use them as gargles, washes, lotions, teas, tinctures (generally stronger than teas and usually diluted with water), ointments, douches, and mouthwashes.

BACK PAIN

Much lower back pain is temporary and nothing seems to cure it better than rest. If there's any inflammation of the area, apply cold packs. Then, after the swelling subsides, heat may be used to keep the muscles relaxed. Most doctors recommend that you not stay down constantly with minor back pain, as the muscles can weaken and further complicate the problem.

St.-John's-wort. This herb has a direct healing action on nerve tissue and is sometimes nicknamed *chiropractor in a bottle.* Gently rub it onto the affected area of the back or neck for extra healing relief. Drink doses of St.-John's-wort to help heal the nerves from within.

Tea. Invariably, when my back hurts, I have been doing too much running around for everyone but myself. It is my body's way of making me take the time to slow down, calm, and relax (whether I think I can or not). Drinking lemon balm or rose petal tea helps add the dimension of taking care of myself back into my routine.

Poplar bark. Drink infusions of poplar bark to ease pain and inflammation. But be careful — pain is nature's way of telling you to rest. Pain-diminishing herbs are best used when you know you will be taking it easy, not to allow you to keep on going until real damage is done.

BLEEDING, CUTS, AND SCRAPES

To control bleeding from a wound, elevate the injured part and, with a clean cloth, press directly on the wound. Keep pressing until the bleeding stops. If the bleeding is serious, do not take the pressure away to brew a cup of tea or powder an herb. Instead maintain pressure and seek medical attention.

White or black walnut bark tea. This will act as a styptic to stanch the flow of blood from a cut. Compresses of the strong tea are most effective.

Peppermint leaf. Finely powdered, this will immediately help clot blood; it's especially helpful to control nosebleeds and razor cuts. For nosebleeds, tilt head back and pinch the nose firmly until the bleeding stops. Use only small amounts of the powdered leaf. I remember being hesitant to try this, worried that it would sting or, by adding "'debris" to the cut, make it worse. It does neither, as long as the peppermint is finely powdered. Try it on a small paper cut first if you are unsure.

Red raspberry leaf. This can be drunk during pregnancy and delivery to help prevent uterine hemorrhaging.

Astringent herbs. Herbs such as lavender, rose, and inner poplar bark made into an infusion are excellent for washing the debris from scrapes.

Garlic wine. See instructions for making this on page 63; it will simultaneously cleanse and prevent infection in wounds and cuts. To protect area after cleansing, apply a paste of garlic honey over areas larger than a quarter, or white pine sap over areas smaller than a quarter as a protective bandage.

St.-John's-wort oil. This will help stimulate the nerve endings for rapid healing. Be sure the cut is clean, as the new skin may grow over dirt and infection.

BOILS AND ABSCESSES

Applications of warm washcloths may be all that is needed to bring a boil or abscess to a head. If it occurs in the breast of a nursing woman, have her continue nursing or expressing milk during treatment, and monitor for signs of mastitis. (These include fever, the area becoming hot to the touch, and nauseous flulike symptoms. Medical treatment may be necessary.)

Honey. This is one of the oldest and simplest remedies for stubborn boils. It can be applied directly to raise the boil; for best results, leave on overnight.

Plantain. Help bring a boil to a head by applying freshly bruised (or chewed) plantain leaf or root to the area. Bind with a cloth and repeat several times a day. Mullein root, mallow root, and violet leaf may be used in a similar manner.

Thyme. Dip a cloth in a cup of strong, warm thyme tea. Apply this compress for ten to fifteen minutes at a time, remoistening the cloth in the warm tea as it cools. Do this several times a day as necessary.

BRUISES

Soothing herbs. Compresses, poultices, or fresh herbs can be simply applied directly to the skin. Use soothing herbs such as lemon balm, mallow root, plantain, violet, walnut leaf, and borage leaf. Add the strong tea to a bath for larger areas. Ointments made from any of these soothing herbs can be spread on afterward to speed healing and relieve discomfort.

Burdock. Drink burdock root tea to help the lymph system heal the bruise from within. You can also wrap the area with large fresh burdock leaves to cool and reduce swelling. Replace with fresh leaves as they become warm and dry.

Mullein. Applications of mullein flower oil are traditionally used in many European households to speed healing and ease painful bruising. The oil is safe enough to use around sensitive areas such as eyelids, mouth, nose, and genitals.

Vinegar. Apply hot or cold compresses of vinegar. Especially helpful are vinegars made with astringent fruits such as blackberry, raspberry, and rose, as they will also help reduce swelling and inflammation.

BUG BITES AND STINGS

For a natural bug repellent, make a smudge by tying together dried lavender, peppermint, mullein, or catnip into a tight cylindrical bundle with thin wire. Light the bundle and keep it nearby. The smoke from the smudge masks your scent and the CO_2 being released with your breath, making it difficult for insects to find you.

If you're out in the field, treat any bites or stings immediately. Honeybees and some wasps leave their stingers behind. Gently scrape them off. Do not pull, as you'll actually release more poison into the sting. Plants such as plantain, mullein, violet, and red clover blossom soothe quickly. Actually, the chlorophyll found in any nonpoisonous green plant will provide relief. Simply rub the juice from the freshly crushed (or chewed) plant on the area. Keep it dirt-free to prevent infection.

Once at home, clean the site well with an antiseptic herb wash such as lavender or thyme, and apply an ice pack to reduce swelling.

For anyone with a large number of insect bites and stings, help the body break down the toxins with herb teas such as oat straw, dandelion root, red clover, and burdock root.

A smudge bundle is a natural bug repellent.

BEWARE BUG BITE ALLERGIES

Always watch for signs of an allergic reaction. About one person in two hundred has a latent severe allergic response because their immune system has been sensitized by a previous bite. A subsequent bite — even years later — may trigger a response that leads to shock and possibly death. Emergency medical intervention is required when:

- ◆ There is swift localized swelling
- ◆ The person was stung in the throat or the mouth
- ◆ Swallowing or breathing becomes difficult
- ◆ The face, lips, eyes, or tongue swells
- ◆ Nausea, vomiting, stomach cramps, or diarrhea occurs
- ◆ The person is dizzy or collapses

BURNS AND BLISTERS

Do not try to treat third-degree burns, burns over a large area of the body, or chemical or electrical burns at home. Instead, stabilize the person, monitor for shock, and arrange transport or emergency medical treatment immediately. I have, however, treated severe second-degree burns when necessity demanded it.

First, assess the situation and remove the person from any further danger. If it is a chemical burn, keep flushing the skin with cold running water until well after the pain has stopped. Keep foremost in mind the importance of not damaging the skin any further, and keep the burn as clean as possible. Clean the area of any debris or dirt very gently — do not break any skin or blistered areas. For first- and mild second-degree burns, immediately place the area in cold water to ease the pain, as long as the skin is not broken.

Vitamin E. There has been much research done showing the efficacy of vitamin E oil to heal burns. The oil works in three ways: It rapidly heals damaged nerve endings; it attracts dead skin cells that are being sloughed off naturally, acting as a natural skin graft; and it acts as an antioxidant to prevent infection.

Salve. A combination of St.-John's-wort and poplar made into a salve with vitamin E (rose hip seeds are a good source) will add the dimension of pain and inflammation relief and nerve fiber rejuvenation to a remedy. Smear the area liberally with the salve. Bandage, changing the dressing two or three times a day until signs of healing are obvious. New skin may grow back fused together, so wrap digits individually. Monitor for any signs of infection, and seek treatment if the area shows any signs of worsening.

White pine sap. If you're in the field, you can re-create the effects of the salve with white pine sap. The Ojibway always made sure there was a white pine tree (or balsam fir, tamarack, or spruce) right next to the fires in their maple sugar camps to heal the inevitable burns and blisters. Reserve straight white pine sap for field use or smaller burns, as it will attract a lot of dirt to its surface. This is fine for small areas, as the dirt can be contained; as the old sap falls off of larger areas, though, the possibility of contaminating the burn increases. Do not remove the old sap; instead, simply cover the area with new sap until healing is complete. When we were camping, my two-year-old son placed his palm on a hot woodstove. His moderate to severe second-degree burns healed without complications or scars, using only constant applications of white pine sap. I've had similar results using balsam fir or balsam poplar bud resins.

> ### DO HERBAL SALVES HEAL?
>
> Once, out of curiosity as to whether it was the salve itself that heals or the herbs in the salve, I experimented on a case of diaper rash. On one area, I applied a plain jojoba and beeswax salve; on the other I used the same plain salve as a base, but augmented it with infused plantain and lemon balm. Would I surprise you if I said that the herbal salve healed overnight, while the plain salve took a week to heal? I hope not, because that's what happened.

Tea. Give the burned person plenty of fluids. A tea made from poplar and lemon balm will help calm the patient and provide a further measure of pain relief.

Salves for sunburn. For sunburn and mild burns, cool the area with cold water or a vinegar splash, then apply a soothing and healing salve. Salves from violet, poplar, rose, lavender, red clover, or plantain will prove helpful.

Mallow root. Cook mallow root until the liquid resembles a gooey egg white, allow to cool, and apply to large areas of minor sunburn. Once the sunburn starts to heal, mix this with an equal amount of thick oat water for relief from itching.

Make oat water as you would any other simple tea, using 1 ounce of rolled oats as the herb to 1 quart of water. Strain and cool before using.

CHAPPED SKIN

Oats. Fill a muslin bag with oats, tie it, and add it to your bathwater; or rub it over the chapped area several times daily.

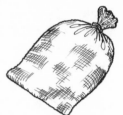

Healing salve. Spread a soothing, healing salve over the affected area. Add extra beeswax, lanolin, coconut oil, or cocoa butter, for a thicker, longer-lasting salve. Infused plaintain and lemon balm are healing additions (see box on page 87). Other helpful herbs to use are violet leaf, mullein leaf or root, mallow leaf or root, red clover blossom, and St.-John's-wort leaf. Avoid applying honey or white pine pitch to chapped skin — it will dry the skin further.

COLDS AND COUGHS

Mild herbal tea. One of the nice things about herbal teas is the amount of water they encourage you to drink. I have quite literally drunk colds away. I'll brew up a pot of whatever mild and nourishing herb I have and drink, drink,

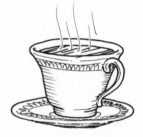

drink . . . as much as a quart an hour if I feel really foul. Make the tea pleasant to taste, rather than medicinal, so you can drink large amounts. Try teas made from rose hips or petal, alfalfa, borage leaf, catnip, dandelion, fresh lemon balm, peppermint, red clover, strawberry leaf or flower or fruit, violet leaf or flower . . . you get the idea.

Baths. Combine the previous tea therapy with hot foot- or full baths of ginger or peppermint to induce perspiration and eliminate body toxins. This can also reduce head congestion by drawing blood away from the head and into the feet.

Mullein leaf. An infusion of fresh or dried mullein leaf is the prime remedy for easing bronchial complaints, hacking or spastic coughs, and lung complaints. To offset its tannin content, boil the leaves in milk for 10 minutes, then strain through a cloth to remove the tiny leaf hairs.

Some people prefer to smoke mullein and substitute mullein leaf for tobacco in hand-rolled cigarettes or light the leaves in a stone dish and inhale the smoke. Smoking mullein has the same effect as drinking a mullein infusion, only the action is faster. And as with any remedy, the faster the action, the greater chance for harm: In this case, though the medicine is healing, the method used (smoking) may be irritating. However, I have successfully used mullein smoke to instantly stop dangerous whooping cough spasms and mild asthma attacks, and I certainly prefer it to the side effects that come from using the medication in over-the-counter and prescription inhalers.

Honey. Take a teaspoon of fresh honey for immediate relief from irritating tickle coughs. Make a honey syrup from violet blossom, borage leaf, crushed garlic clove, mallow root, plantain leaf, red clover blossom, thyme, or white pine needle. All have expectorant or emollient properties.

Garlic. Garlic's reputation for healing bronchial and lung complaints is well deserved. I have seen it cure chronic bronchitis that antibiotics could not touch. Adding a fresh clove of garlic a day to the diet can prevent asthma attacks and reverse that disease's deadly downward spiral. Eat a sprig of parsley or dandelion leaf afterward to help control garlic's odor.

Pine. Pour a quart of boiling water over a good handful of fresh pine needles, place a towel over your head and the pine tea, and breathe deeply of its vapors to break up congestion quickly. When finished, strain and drink the beverage to get high doses of vitamins C and A to further speed your recovery. Adding a little lemon and honey will make the beverage more enjoyable.

For herbal therapies that help the body's immune system combat cold viruses, see the section on flu prevention.

CONSTIPATION

Constipation is usually caused by not eating enough fruits, vegetables, or foods with natural fiber, or by lack of exercise. The safest remedy may be as simple as drinking several glasses of water and enjoying a walk.

Strawberry. This fruit has a mild laxative effect, and is especially useful when the constipation is due to excessive meats or fats in the diet.

Mullein. Mullein tea made with milk will help a person pass hard stools easier because of its demulcent and emollient properties.

Greens. Intensely green leaves are slightly laxative to many people. Add servings of fresh or steamed violet leaf, dandelion greens, or plantain leaf to the diet. This has the added benefit of replacing possible lost nutrients.

Honey. This also has a slight laxative effect.

Plaintain. Pour a cup of boiling water over 1 tablespoon of coarsely ground plantain seeds. Let sit for 20 minutes and drink, without straining, just before bedtime. This is an excellent laxative for more persistent constipation, or constipation from pregnancy, iron supplements, or prescribed medication. The seeds replace valuable B vitamins, soothe the entire digestive tract, and have no known harmful chemical or drug interactions. Do not use, however, if you have diverticulosis, as the seeds may cause irritation.

CRAMPS AND SPASMS

Calcium. Frequent muscle spasms and cramping are often an indication of too little calcium in the diet. Drink teas rich in calcium such as dandelion, oat straw, raspberry, and plantain leaf. Common foods rich in calcium include almonds, carob, sesame seeds, yogurt, and most deep green vegetables.

Lavender. Lavender is both antispasmodic and sedative. Drink as a tea, or apply directly to the area as a wash or poultice for direct relief.

HOMEMADE CALCIUM SUPPLEMENT

Make your own daily calcium supplement by filling a jar halfway with organic crushed eggshells. Cover with vinegar and let sit for 2 weeks. Strain, then take 1 to 3 tablespoons daily. You can use this as salad dressing, in sauces, or sweetened with honey for a refreshing beverage, so you don't feel like it's medicine.

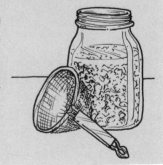

Mullein leaf. When smoked, mullein can instantly relax the bronchial spasms associated with asthma, whooping cough, and bronchitis.

Ginger. Drink ginger tea to relieve either stomach or menstrual cramping.

DETOXIFICATION

Dandelion and burdock root. If you buy an herbal detoxification formula, chances are its prime ingredients will be either dandelion or burdock root. But why buy it when you can get the fresh root for free? They are used worldwide whenever liver-related problems are involved. Both promote kidney function, too, and have abundant minerals to replace any that may be eliminated in urine. Dandelion tremendously benefits the digestive system, while burdock excels at alleviating chronic skin disorders and eruptions.

Red clover. Daily doses of red clover tea will help reduce the symptoms from steroids, radiation, or chemotherapy. It also has mild blood-thinning capabilities, making it useful as a preventative for arteriosclerosis and high cholesterol.

Thyme. Drink a cup of thyme tea to recover from a wild time. It will ease headache, nervousness, and the queasy stomach of a hangover more effectively and safely than over-the-counter sedatives or pain relievers.

Borage. Borage seed oil helps ease the stress from long-term chronic metabolic disorders such as menopausal distress, alcoholism, obesity, and steroid treatments. It also offers quick relief to a hangover.

DIARRHEA

Diarrhea can quickly become dangerous. If it lasts for more than four days (one day for small children) and is not getting better, if the person vomits everything he drinks or drinks nothing, if there is blood in the stools, or if the person is dehydrated and getting worse, prompt medical attention should be sought.

Rehydrating liquids. Any person with watery diarrhea is in danger of dehydration, especially a child. Do not wait until dehydration begins to start replacing lost fluids. Administer sips of a rehydrating drink every five minutes day and night until urination is normal. For babies, it is best to take the

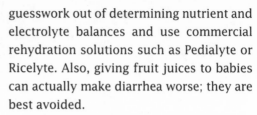

WARNING: BEWARE DEHYDRATION

Any person with diarrhea should be watched carefully for signs of severe dehydration. If the skin becomes loose, cold, or clammy; the eyes sunken and tearless; the urine strong smelling; the mouth dry; or (for babies) the soft spot on the head does not rebound when pressed, seek medical treatment immediately.

guesswork out of determining nutrient and electrolyte balances and use commercial rehydration solutions such as Pedialyte or Ricelyte. Also, giving fruit juices to babies can actually make diarrhea worse; they are best avoided.

Starchy fluids. These are a great cure for diarrhea. Make a thick oatmeal drink by cooking together 1 cup of oats and 2 quarts of water for 5 minutes. Strain and drink frequently in small sips. Starchy fluids tend to diminish vomiting and reduce fluid loss (unlike sweetened sugary drinks and sodas). If possible, make the drink with herbs that have high potassium content, such as alfalfa, borage, clover blossom, dandelion, raspberry, and pine needles.

Blackberry root. This has been the herb of choice to eliminate diarrhea and dysentery throughout history. Make the standard medicinal dose, and drink 1 teaspoon every five minutes until the diarrhea is under control. Repeat as necessary. Its milder cousins, raspberry and rose leaf, may be used in the form of a tea for small children.

Yogurt. This is one of the safest foods you can eat to prevent diarrhea because it is unlikely to have *E. coli* bacteria, the main cause of food poisoning. Eating plain yogurt daily also helps prevent diarrhea, as does drinking vinegar beverages sweetened with honey before meals.

Mullein. Mullein leaf tea is a mild astringent useful to help control diarrhea, especially in children. Add a tablespoon of plain yogurt to the mullein to offset its tannin content and add beneficial bacteria.

EARACHE

Olive oil and garlic. Plain olive oil is a traditional remedy used to soothe earaches quickly. Simply put a few drops of warm olive oil in the ear and have the person rest on their side with the ear up, for about five minutes so the oil has a chance to flow down into the inner ear. If agreeable to the patient, gently massage around the outside of the ear.

For further relief, I'll smash a clove of garlic and let it rest in warm olive oil for fifteen minutes and strain. Then, I'll take a one-inch cotton ball, let it soak up the garlic olive oil and place it so it rests just inside the outer earlobe. The cotton keeps the oil inside the ear, and the garlic helps combat the infection. Now have the patient turn and rest the troubled ear on a heating pad for about thirty minutes. The heat and gravity will help the ear drain, but the cotton will keep the oil from escaping. Repeat as needed, using fresh garlic and cotton each time. If the patient is prone to earaches, taking the above steps at the onset of colds or after swimming helps prevent ear infections in the first place — infinitely preferable to having to fight against an earache.

Always be sure the eardrum is not ruptured before putting anything in the ear. If the earache is persistent or recurring, consult a physician, as deafness may occur. Drink plenty of water, nutritive tonic herbs, and eat wholesome foods to build strength.

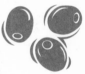

Mullein flower oil. Penelope Ody, a member of the National Institute of Medical Herbalists in the United Kingdom, cites in her book, *The Complete Medicinal Herbal,* the still-current use of mullein flower oil to soothe ear inflammations.

Plaintain. Drink plantain tea to help tone the delicate membranes of the inner ear. It also helps reduce chronic dizziness from ear inflammations.

Food allergies. Suspect food allergies if the ear infections are recurring. One study showed nearly 75 percent of a group of children scheduled to have tubes surgically placed into their ears showed sensitivity to milk, wheat, eggs, peanuts, or soy products. It may take the infections several months to clear up after the food culprit is removed from the diet.

ENERGY-BUILDING TONICS

Traditionally tonic herbs were taken after a steady winter diet of dried, salted, fatty foods. They help rejuvenate the body and bring energy levels up to the high demands placed on it through spring, summer, and harvest chores. Tonics nourish and promote general health of the internal organs, especially the liver, a main detoxifying organ of the body.

Spring tonics. These are usually made from spring's abundant green growth. Sometimes they consist of nothing more than plates of lightly steamed or salad greens such as dandelion greens, young garlic shoots, mallow leaves, and plantain or violet leaves and blossoms. Roots from dandelion or burdock that overwintered can be included for extra detoxifying action and to add depth to the flavor.

Winter tonic. Strawberry leaf tea is a simple old-fashioned wintertime tonic. Abundant in vitamin C, green year-round, strawberry also helps improve circulation to fight off winter's cold from within.

General tonics. Dandelion and burdock roots are two of the best general tonics that nature has to offer us. They may be combined or used separately; fresh, tinctured, or dried; in foods or as medicines; and some form of each is available year-round . . . whew, with flexibility like that no wonder these are so highly esteemed by herbalists around the world!

Blood tonic. Red clover blossom tea is a standard old-time blood tonic, and has often been used in conjunction with other herbs such as violet, burdock, dandelion, and garlic for the treatment of cancer and tumors. Today you'll see it frequently employed to help reduce the serious side effects from radiation and chemotherapy treatments.

MY ALL-AROUND NOURISHING TONIC

Nature has a capricious whimsy that can become a bit of a sore thorn when you start to gather your own plants for medicine. One year may be great for red clover, and then there may not be another good crop for four or five years. It's frustrating to learn about an herb only to be unable to get enough the next year. So rather than rely on one herb, I make what I fondly call my backyard blend.

The blend changes from year to year depending on what nature has grown in abundance and what I've happened to gather. I simply dry the herbs, put them all together in one big paper bag, and grab a handful when I want a cup of nourishing tonic tea. The herbs are always nourishing simples such as red clover, borage leaf and flower, violet, plantain, alfalfa, and rose petal or hips. Unlike an herbal formula tailored to a specific ailment — where you try to keep the variety of herbs to a minimum — in this instance I use as wide a variety of simple foodlike herbs as possible, to get a broad spectrum of vitamins and minerals and to create a general nourishing tonic.

EYES

Rub your palms together briskly until they are quite warm. Now press your palms to your eyes for quick relief from eye strain, tiredness, and slight twitches.

Cool compresses. Soothe hot, inflamed eyes by placing cool compresses of plantain, lemon balm, or rose water on them. Let rest for five minutes at a time. This also can be used to clean away excessive eye mucus from conjunctivitis or pink eye.

Borage. Borage leaf was much valued by the ancient Greeks for strengthening weak eyes and preventing cataracts. Recent studies show you are eleven times more likely to develop cataracts if your diet lacks in beta-carotene, folic acid, and vitamin C. Borage has plenty, as do many other dark leafy greens such as dandelion and violet.

FEVERS

Fever is the way the body kick-starts the immune system, and it may not be necessary to do anything but give the patient rest and plenty of fluids, and let nature take her course. Generally, this holds true if the fever stays under 100°F and lasts for no more than 2–3 days. Water is fever's nemesis. Flush the fever from the body by having the patient drink plenty of soothing and pleasant-tasting herb teas such as lemon balm, mallow-violet, rose hip, and lavender, or plain water.

Fruit teas. As a fever mounts, digestion slows. Avoid eating foods that are hard to digest. Instead drink mild, cooling fruit teas such as strawberry, raspberry vinegar, or rose petal tea.

Poplar bark. This should *not* be used to relieve fevers, aches, and pains in young children, as it contains the chemical precursor to aspirin and may cause complications. It may, however, be safely used by adults in combination with an emollient herb such as mallow or plantain.

SOOTHING BABY'S MINOR EYE IRRITATIONS

Nursing mothers have the perfect remedy for baby's minor eye irritations and inflammations. Simply use a squirt of breast milk as a soothing wash. Breast milk is sterile as it leaves the breast, warm, and soothing; it also contains the mother's natural antibodies to help ward off infection.

WARNING

A fever that continues to rise or rises rapidly may be an indication of a systemic bacterial infection. Seek immediate medical treatment.

Borage. A cup of strong, warm borage lemonade will cool a fever while stimulating the kidneys to flush poisons from the system. The high vitamin and mineral content will help the person regain strength.

Encourage sweating. Burdock, catnip, ginger, and peppermint encourage sweating, and may be used as teas or baths to help break moderate fevers.

To bring down a fever, frequently sponge the patient's neck, forehead, ears, armpits, groin, and soles of feet with tepid brews of peppermint, catnip, or ginger. Have the patient drink as much water as possible, but in small frequent sips. Administer a teaspoon to a tablespoon of peppermint, catnip, or ginger tea every five minutes until the fever lowers.

FLU PREVENTION

The best prevention against viral infections is the resounding good health that comes from adding fresh herbs to your daily diet. Growing up in a medical family, and later working in a restaurant, I have been able to witness firsthand how easily germs are spread. Keeping your hands away from your eyes, nose, and mouth and washing them frequently will go a long way toward ensuring that the season's flu passes you by.

Garlic. Add 1 to 2 cloves of fresh raw garlic into your daily diet. Fresh garlic can be sprinkled on top of salads, soups, or bread, or mixed with honey, to help minimize possible stomach upsets.

Thyme. This herb has potent antiviral and antibiotic qualities. Start drinking thyme as your daily beverage when everyone around you is getting the flu. If it is too late and you are already ill, thyme tea will lesson the duration and severity of the illness.

Rose hips. These are one of nature's best sources of vitamin C, and complement the flavor of nearly every herb you may choose to use to prevent colds and flus. Other herbs that are a good source of vitamins C or A are alfalfa, catnip, lemon balm, plantain, strawberry leaf, violet leaf, and white pine needle.

Violet. The common violet acts as a gentle immune-system stimulant. Drink a tea made from the whole aboveground portion of the plant. Other herbs that help stimulate the immune system to combat viral infections are St.-John's-wort, white pine, and strawberry leaf.

Yogurt. Plain yogurt can kill bacteria all on its own, but it will also help your body gear up for production of antibodies to kill invading organisms.

FROSTBITE

Mullein. Topical applications of mullein flower oil speed recovery from frostbite.

Mallow root. Make a warm mash of equal amounts of mallow root and oatmeal. Apply as a paste to the affected parts to help hold the heat to the area, and to soothe and protect.

Peppermint. Drink a tea made from equal amounts of peppermint and young strawberry leaf to help improve overall circulation.

Ginger. A salve made from peppermint or ginger can be applied before going out into cold conditions for long periods of time. The oil will protect the skin while the herb brings the blood to the area, thus helping to prevent frostbite. Small amounts of powdered ginger may also be simply sprinkled directly into your shoes.

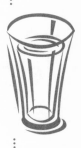

Plenty of water. One of the secrets the most successful mountain climbers have is to drink copious amounts of water, because during extremely cold weather, the body loses a lot of moisture. If you know you'll be outside for an extended period of time, drink plenty of water, avoid consuming alcohol, and wear protective layered clothing.

GRAY HAIR

Folklore gives us many ways to prevent gray hair, and research lends credibility to some of the claims. Studies show that a diet lacking in any one of the following nutrients (they're all in the B vitamin group) produces lack of hair pigmentation, resulting in gray hair: folic acid, pantothenic acid, biotin, and para-amino-benzoic acid (PABA).

Unfortunately, the corresponding corollary that a diet rich in these nutrients reverses graying hair isn't quite accurate. Genetic tendencies and individual needs mean that what works for the goose doesn't always work for the gander. Folic acid seems to be the most effective nutrient in reversing gray hair. Biotin comes in a close second, but sometimes a combination of the two, or three, or even all four nutrients is needed. And some hair will remain gray no matter what nutrients are added to the diet. There is no doubt, however, that these nutrients play a strong role in determining the color and health of your hair.

Although the most concentrated doses of these nutrients are found in the organ meats, notably liver and kidneys, the plant world has good sources also.

Folic acid. The term *folic acid* is derived from the word *foliage.* It is abundant in most dark leafy greens. You will find it in the spinachlike herbs plantain, mallow, violet, dandelion, and alfalfa, and also in flavorful lemon balm, catnip, peppermint, and red clover. (The roots contain little folic acid.)

Plantain seeds are an excellent source of easily assimilated B vitamins, and I have met several people who swear they owe their abundant dark hair (and the fact that lice, ticks, and mosquitoes leave them alone) to sprinkling crushed plantain seeds on each meal.

Italians claim to look young with dandelion flower wine and green salads that contain solid levels of all four B vitamins.

Black walnut coloring. Meanwhile, to cover up the gray, make an infusion from the hulls of the black walnut, and dab it on the gray spots for a deep brown color that stays for about four to six weeks and lasts even through daily shampooing.

HEADACHE

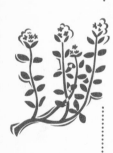

Headaches (except for certain kinds of migraine headaches) are a symptom, not an illness in themselves. An estimated 90 percent of intermittent headaches stem from stress, eyestrain, colds and flus, dehydration, or fatigue. Once again, the classic remedy of rest and drinking plenty of fluids is bound to help. However, some headaches are due to inactivity. Simply step outside, breathe deeply, and go for a walk.

Calming teas. Drink calming and soothing teas such as catnip, lemon balm, lavender, rose petal, and violet. Or add them to a warm bath and let the water soak away your tension.

If the tension is concentrated in one area, apply hot compresses or a hot-water bottle to the area during the bath.

Rub the temples. Use an infusion or ointment made from lavender, peppermint, thyme, or ginger for tension headaches. Likewise, for sinus headaches, rub the sinus cavities with these warming herbs to help break up congestion.

Ginger. A daily drink of ginger has been shown to be nearly as effective at preventing migraines as powerful prescription drugs, with none of the debilitating side effects. Ginger oil can be rubbed onto the temples during early warning signs to thwart the oncoming migraine completely. To relieve pressure, soak your feet in a hot footbath with ginger or peppermint added to it. The bath draws the blood away from the head to the heat and provides a measure of relief.

Exhaustion. For headaches from nervous exhaustion, drink strong teas of alfalfa, St.-John's-wort, borage, or oat straw.

Poplar bark. An infusion of poplar bark will relieve most headaches in a manner similar to aspirin's. Combine with mallow root to ease possible stomach upset. (**Caution:** As with aspirin, poplar should *not* be taken by children with a high fever.)

WARNING

Chronic headaches may be an indication of severe problems. If the headache persists, bring it to the attention of a health professional.

HEART PROBLEMS

Any heart trouble is potentially deadly serious and a health professional should be consulted at signs of trouble. However, simple herbs have a remarkable ability to keep trouble from arising in the first place.

Garlic. This remarkable plant is accepted as beneficial to the heart by both traditional and modern medicine. Garlic reduces cholesterol, reduces the buildup of fatty deposits in the arteries, lowers blood pressure, and helps prevent blood clots from forming — with no harmful side effects, and as effectively as some pharmaceutical drugs! Research shows that garlic may even prevent a second heart attack if you've had one already. The good news is that the compounds that give garlic its circulatory benefits are present in its every form: fresh, cooked, dried, and even powdered.

Use homemade preparations of garlic whenever possible. You will save tremendous amounts of money. Also, the main reason most people use capsules is to reduce the odor of garlic — but if the odor is missing, so are the many benefits of garlic.

Wine. If alcohol presents no problem to you, statistical evidence shows that drinking a glass of red wine before dinner will reduce the risk of heart attack by as much as 30 percent! Red wines seem to be slightly more beneficial than white. Home-made wines with herbs that enhance circulation, such as red clover, will add an extra benefit. However, even moderate alcohol consumption may bring on chest pain if you have angina, and those who drink more than a glass a day are putting themselves at risk for other health problems.

Oats. Three decades of research confirms the power of oatmeal to drive down cholesterol. All it takes is 2 ounces of oat bran a day, or ⅔ cup of oatmeal. Oats have a soluble gummy fiber that helps prevent cholesterol from being absorbed during digestion and thus keeps it from entering the bloodstream.

Walnuts. Even though walnuts are high in fat, it is a type of fat that helps lower cholesterol! In an otherwise low-fat diet, eating a few nuts a day (2 ounces) can help reduce cholesterol levels as much as 18 percent.

Vitamins and minerals. Eating fruits and vegetables rich in vitamin C, beta carotene, potassium, and vitamin E can help detoxify bad cholesterol and lower high blood pressure. Some of the twenty-five basic herbs used in this book (see pages 26–37) that are good sources are alfalfa, borage, catnip, dandelion, lemon balm, mallow leaves, peppermint, plantain, red clover, rose hips, strawberry, raspberry, violet, and white pine needle.

Red clover has a special compound called coumarin that helps thin the blood and prevent clotting. Combine with alfalfa to receive ample amounts of the vitamins and minerals that strengthen blood vessel walls.

HEMORRHOIDS

Hemorrhoids are varicose veins of the rectum. They may be painful but generally are not dangerous. They frequently appear during pregnancy, or may indicate poor nutrition. It helps to eat plenty of fruit, leafy greens, and foods with a lot of fiber (such as oats) to prevent constipation and rebuild the strength of the delicate membranes.

Astringent plant juices. Dabbing the juice of one of these plants on the hemorrhoids will help shrink them: blackberry leaf, poplar bark, raspberry leaf, or rose leaf or bark. These are all strong astringents.

Mullein. Mullein flower oil will help relieve pain and itching from external hemorrhoids.

INDIGESTION

Antacids are two of the top ten items purchased in grocery stores across America! TV commercials have convinced us that the cause of our indigestion is too much acid; actually, however, the average person has too *little* acid. A healthy person's stomach manufactures a strong acid called hydrochloric acid (HCL). As we become older, our diet deficient, or our life stressful, our body produces less and less HCL. Taking antacids often starts a vicious downspiral in which more and more are needed to prevent indigestion, while our food is actually not being digested at all! Symptoms of too little acid can be exactly the same as those of too much. Do not use antacid tablets until you have *confirmed* you really do have an overacid stomach.

Slow down and chew. We are always in such a hurry that we gulp through our meals, rush off to the next project, and complain when our stomachs rebel. Simply taking the time to enjoy your meal, chew your food, and savor the flavor is all the "medicine" it may take to eliminate indigestion altogether.

Sweetened vinegar. If you are lacking in stomach acid, the simplest way to add acid to your diet is with sweetened vinegar beverages. Simply put 1 tablespoon in a cup of water, sweeten with honey, and drink the tea ten to fifteen minutes before eating your meal.

Yogurt. Because of the high use of broad-spectrum antibiotics in this country, indigestion may be caused by a lack of beneficial intestinal bacteria. A sure remedy is to eat at least a cup of plain yogurt or other cultured milk such as kefir and acidophilus each day.

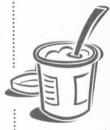

Mint. Few plants aid digestion in as pleasant a way as mint. Though we are familiar with mint in candies, ice creams, jams, and even cigarettes, these commercial products use mint extracts, which just cannot compete with the wonderful flavor and fragrance of fresh-picked green mint. Simply smelling fresh peppermint makes my mouth water and stirs up my appetite. Added to a salad (as is done throughout the Near East), it makes a wonderful meal starter that keeps indigestion from occurring at all. When the mint is blended with other greens, vegetables, and oil and vinegar, it does not overpower the salad as you may think, but instead simply adds a freshness to the whole spectrum of flavors.

Mint tea is a worldwide favorite remedy for upset stomach, nausea, flatulence, and weak appetite. It is safe enough for very small children — though they may prefer the milder flavor of spearmint.

Ginger. Ginger tea generally brings more warmth to stimulate digestion than does mint. The flavor is generally preferred by adults; also, strong ginger can cause unpleasant hiccupping and belching in small children. Sucking on a piece of candied ginger is an alternative. Ginger is especially beneficial after a heavy meal.

Catnip. Cold catnip tea can be drunk before meals to stimulate appetite, and warm catnip tea drunk after meals to prevent gas. Catnip makes a pleasantly refreshing beverage, and was the beverage of choice for much of Europe before the introduction of Oriental tea. A slice of lemon enhances its flavor perfectly. Catnip is excellent for calming a nervous stomach. Traditionally, teas made from red clover or catnip were drunk to soothe and heal irritated stomach ulcers.

Thyme. Thyme tea is a classic remedy for the stomach chills or upsets associated with colds and flus.

INFANT AILMENTS

Infants and babies are especially vulnerable to complications from both illness and treatment. Always choose the least amount of intervention necessary to alleviate any problem. When using herbs, remember that they are medicine. Choose extremely mild herbs, such as catnip, spearmint, and oat straw, and make the tea weak by diluting it. Use one part standard infusion to three parts water for babies over three months old.

In most cases when a baby is ill, breast-feeding should be encouraged to continue. Indeed, an ideal way to administer simple herb teas is to have the mother drink the tea and let the baby receive the medicine indirectly through the breast milk.

Colic. Weak catnip tea is the surest remedy for infantile colic. It quiets the nervous system and eases gastric distress. Either the nursing mother can drink the tea and the baby receive it through her milk, or a warm poultice of catnip can be laid on the baby's stomach, or an eyedropperful of the tea can be squirted directly into the baby's mouth. Frequent colic may indicate a food sensitivity — perhaps to cabbage or to cow's milk — which may occur even if the nursing mother is the one eating the allergy-causing foods.

Umbilical stump. Paint a newborn's umbilical stump with honey to prevent infection and help it dry up quickly.

Diaper rash and cradle cap. An infusion of violet, lavender, or plantain tea can be used as a wash for diaper rash or cradle cap.

INFLAMMATIONS AND INFECTIONS

Mallow. Apply poultices of mallow root or mallow leaf to draw out infections and soothe inflamed tissues. Apply the poultice as hot as is tolerable, and then add a hot-water bottle or hot cloth on top to keep it warm. Renew the materials as they cool. Continue this treatment until relief is felt. This remedy works equally well with plantain leaves.

When my husband awoke to a wound with ugly red streaks radiating from a throbbing armpit (indicating blood poisoning), the doctor was unable to see him for several hours. So I treated it as above, and within an hour the swelling had noticeably improved, the throbbing decreased. By the time of the appointment, the red streaks were hardly noticeable, so we canceled and kept up the treatment. By morning the wound itself was nearly healed.

Red clover. Red clover blossom tea will help in all manner of internal inflammations, as it aids the functioning of the lymphatic system. It is equally useful for skin swellings and inflammations, especially arthritic swellings, gout, and external ulcers.

Arthritis. To help prevent arthritis flare-ups, drink alfalfa tea daily.

Violet. Violet poultices will soothe inflamed skin sores and abscesses, as well as help to draw out stubborn infections.

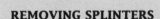

REMOVING SPLINTERS

Paul Kenwaubekesie, who grew up fishing Lake Michigan for a living, taught me this trick to draw out stubborn splinters.

Heat pine pitch until it is warm but still tolerable to be put on the skin. Place the warm pitch on the splinter and let rest until it cools to about skin temperature. Peel off. Usually the splinter comes out on the first try, but you can repeat as needed. Paul used this method to get out stubborn fish spines and scales, just like his grandfather before him.

ITCHING

Vinegar. To relieve itching, try compresses of lukewarm diluted vinegar (¼ cup vinegar per quart of water). Herbal vinegars such as plantain, violet, rose, and lavender will add an extra measure of relief.

Oats. For itching over large areas of skin, put 1 cup of oats in a muslin bag, tie it shut, and toss the bag into a lukewarm bath. The bag can later be remoistened and rubbed over specific areas.

Plaintain. Poultices of plantain or marsh mallow give relief. Simply dip the leaf in warm water to soften it, then bind it to the area with a cloth. Replace when the leaf no longer feels cool.

The skin wash tincture on page 42 works well when itching is due to poison ivy, parasites, or fungal infections. For a simple remedy, try washing with walnut leaf infusion.

Chronic eczema and psoriasis. If the itching is due to a chronic condition such as eczema, topical applications may provide symptom relief but will not address the cause. The skin is a major eliminative organ. When constant eruptions occur on the skin we must look to aid the internal eliminative organs — the kidneys, plus the major detoxifying organ, the liver. Daily doses of infused borage oil are sometimes all that is needed to prevent psoriasis and eczema flare-ups. Adding dandelion to the diet and medicinal doses of dandelion tea will aid both liver and kidney function. Burdock root (used as food or medicine) is most effective for enhancing liver function.

For long-term treatment of acne, eczema, ectopic skin, or psoriasis, a daily tea of burdock root, red clover blossom, and violet leaf is especially helpful. First simmer the burdock root for 10 minutes, then remove from the heat and add the violet leaf and red clover blossom.

KIDNEY AND BLADDER FUNCTION

Yogurt. Eating a cup of yogurt daily to prevent yeast and bladder infections may sound like an old wives' tale, but it really works. The culture must be live to have any effect. For extra relief, add a cup of yogurt to a warm bath, or douche with a tablespoon of yogurt mixed in a quart of warm water.

Burdock and dandelion. Both of these herbs gently stimulate the kidneys to increase the flow of urine, yet have enough vitamins and minerals to replace any that may then be excreted in the urine. Thus they are generally considered safe for long-term use. Dandelion has a greater capacity for clearing obstructions from the kidneys and bladder, while burdock eases the strain on the kidneys by promoting sweat and encouraging the skin to eliminate toxins as well.

Bladder infections. These are the second most common complaint (next to menstrual difficulties) of women. Frequently they coincide with ovulation or pregnancy. Underwear traps bacteria and moisture and creates an ideal breeding ground. Wear none, or wear loose-fitting cotton underwear that breathes, if you are prone to infection. Also, drink copious amounts of water to dilute bacteria concentrations and increase urination; this helps the body rid itself of the bacteria. Avoid caffeine, as it irritates the kidneys; mild diuretics such as dandelion or burdock root help, though. Drinking ½ to 2 cups of cranberry or blueberry juice incapacitates the *E. coli* bacteria responsible for causing the infection. Drink ½ cup daily as a preventative or increase to 2 cups daily to help combat a current infection.

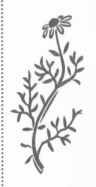

A tea made from equal parts of mallow root, dandelion root, and plantain leaf will relieve kidney and bladder infections. Plantain, especially, helps the kidneys secrete uric acid and is therefore helpful in attacks of gout.

Whenever administering an herb to increase the flow of urine, I add a demulcent herb such as mallow to help soothe any irritated tissue and to ease the possible passage of stones.

Sluggish kidneys. Compresses of warm ginger applied to the abdomen help stimulate sluggish kidneys, without necessarily increasing urine output.

Kidney stones. Drinking daily infusions of rose hip tea has been demonstrated to be useful in preventing and breaking up kidney stones.

MENSTRUATION AND PREGNANCY

It is no coincidence that a highly processed, high-fat diet lacking in fresh vitamins and minerals and menstrual difficulties go hand in hand. Although we have come to accept menstrual cramps, heavy or irregular bleeding, migraines, hot flashes, PMS, and mood swings as normal, they are indications that the body is not able to balance its hormonal cycle in a healthy manner. If you look carefully at most women's herb formulas, they are really nutritional supplements. Commonly used herbs such as dandelion, motherwort, raspberry leaf, burdock root, and nettle are powerhouses of easily assimilated vitamins and minerals.

Diet. Before addressing any symptoms of menstrual distress, look to your overall diet. Are you eating ample amounts of *fresh* fruits and vegetables? Are they organically grown? Do you eat store-bought meat and dairy products, most of which contain low-level amounts of antibiotics and hormonal supplements and so have a disruptive influence on your own hormonal cycle? Do you eat fresh whole grains? Every step you take toward eating good wholesome food is a step toward achieving a balanced cycle.

Borage. Borage seed oil will help the adrenals move stagnant energy in the body and relieve chronic menstrual difficulties such as PMS and difficult menopause. Sprinkle your food with alfalfa or plantain seeds or sprouts to add valuable B vitamins.

Strawberry. Drink strawberry leaf tea daily over a long period of time to regulate the menstrual cycle.

Ginger. Ginger tea and warm ginger poultices will ease menstrual cramping and nausea.

PREGNANCY TONIC

My favorite tonic to ensure a healthy pregnancy consists of equal parts of raspberry leaf, alfalfa leaf, lemon balm, and plantain leaf. I drank this daily when I was carrying my twins, who were born to term. One weighed 7 pounds, 10 ounces, the other 8 pounds, 6 ounces — 16 pounds of baby altogether!

When a friend's rabbits had infertility problems, I suggested she add some of this tea to their water, and her rabbits bred like — well, rabbits. Since then, several women who previously could not conceive or carry a baby to term have tried this tea blend, and are now proud mothers (though that is no actual proof the herbs were responsible). It is primarily a nutritive formula; the raspberry leaf helps strengthen the uterus, the lemon balm eases stress, and the plantain adds internal soothing.

Warming herbs. Other warming stimulant herbs such as peppermint, catnip, and thyme (it isn't called mother of thyme for nothing) can be tried. Also, supplement the diet with herbs high in calcium such as alfalfa, dandelion, and red clover.

Menstrual flow. To control excessive menstrual flow, drink strong teas of red raspberry leaf or red rose petal.

To promote delayed menstruation, a cup of lemon balm tea may be all that is needed to help the person relax and flow with her cycle. In China, ginger tea has been traditionally used to bring on menstruation. This has led to much controversy over the use of ginger in another traditional manner — to help control morning sickness when pregnant. However, studies are showing that ginger used in food or as beverage teas to help control morning sickness is not harmful to pregnancy.

PMS. Ease PMS irritability magically with a bowl of oatmeal! The complex carbohydrates found in oatmeal (and other whole grains) work nearly as well as Valium in calming PMS tension, and the nourishing action of oats calms the nervous system.

MOUTH, GUMS, AND TEETH

Gum tissue. To maintain healthy gums while brushing your teeth, use a homemade toothbrush fashioned from the twig of the walnut, poplar, or rose. This will help tighten your gum tissues, reduce any inflammation, and have a mild antiseptic action. Simply sharpen one end of a pencil-length twig to use as a toothpick and chew on the fibers of the other end to use as a brush. Remove the thorns from the rose first by rubbing the twig lightly with a knife.

Use long rose or blackberry thorns as a field toothpick. Naturally grown thorns are sharper than toothpicks, they hold a point longer, and their curved shape makes them easier to use.

Mouthwash. The simplest mouthwash of all is a fresh, aromatic, antiseptic leaf chewed slowly. Lavender, lemon balm, peppermint, and thyme all excel as mouthwashes.

Tooth whitener. Rub your teeth with a fresh strawberry to whiten them. Diluted strawberry and peppermint tincture makes an excellent antiseptic mouthwash.

Teething. Babies may get relief by chewing on a piece of fresh catnip or peppermint, or the freshly crushed leaf can be rubbed over the area.

Abscess. To relieve an abscessed tooth, rub the area with a fresh garlic clove cut in half, and eat 1 to 2 fresh cloves of garlic daily.

Tooth decay. We all have heard the studies that link tooth decay to sweets. Less known, however, is that poor nutrition is also linked to tooth decay. A diet abundant in minerals gives you the building blocks necessary to maintain healthy, cavity-free teeth. Add liberal amounts of mineral-rich herbs such as alfalfa, burdock, dandelion, and violet to your diet to keep your smile free and easy.

Thrush infections. Chew fresh garlic and eat lots of yogurt to combat thrush infections.

Cold sores. These stem from a viral infection and tend to recur when a person is ill or under stress. The easiest remedy I know of is to keep the sore painted with pure honey until it is healed, and add a little powdered garlic or thyme to speed the healing along.

Mouth sores. Narrow sores at the corners of the mouth are another sign of poor nutrition. Treat them with an antiseptic wash of thyme or lavender and add fresh whole grains, fruits, and vegetables to the diet, while eliminating sweets.

Suck on a pastille made from equal amounts of finely chopped balsam poplar buds and powdered plantain leaf to heal stubborn mouth sores and ulcers. If the sore stems from a viral infection, add an equal amount of powdered lemon balm leaf when making the pastille.

NERVOUSNESS

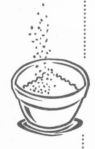

Lavender. A few drops of infused lavender oil or a lavender infusion can be rubbed on the temples to dispel nervous tension. Drinking lavender infusion will enhance the action.

Catnip. If a person has the tendency to place nervous tension in the stomach, infusions of catnip tea will help calm and relax. If there is vomiting, apply a warm poultice of catnip directly onto the stomach.

Oats. Oats and oat straw tea are specifically nourishing to the nerves. Anyone who has difficulty dealing with stress or has chronic nervous tension should be encouraged to eat oats daily.

Lemon balm and rose petals. These both help lighten the heart and lift the spirits. Drink freely and as often as needed.

Poplar bark. To reduce pain from inflamed nerves, apply poultices of poplar bark, or St.-John's-wort oil, directly to the affected area.

Alfalfa. This makes a superlative tonic to speed recovery from nervous exhaustion or burnout, but has an aftertaste that many people do not enjoy. However, if you combine it with equal amounts of borage leaf and lemon balm, it makes a scrumptious lemonade-type beverage.

OVERWEIGHT

Chew well. "Fletcher" your food. In 1898 Horace Fletcher became the spokesperson for thoroughly chewing your food when he lost 60 pounds of fat in five months — with no other changes than chewing his food thoroughly, in a relaxed manner, and eating only when hungry. "Fletcherizing" became all the rage in his day, but studies still show that simply chewing your food to a pulpy liquid does indeed help with weight loss.

Ginger and spice. Eat spicy hot foods to rev up your metabolism and burn off fat. Drinking ginger tea may actually increase metabolism as much as 25 percent, helping you to burn off extra calories.

Digestion herbs. Herbs that aid digestion also help the body eliminate fat. Dandelion is the queen of the fat-burning herbs; mild in action, it will also replace any minerals lost to its slight diuretic action. Other herbs that help are burdock, catnip, lavender, and thyme.

For herbs to help combat fat in the blood (cholesterol and triglycerides), see the section on heart problems.

RECOVERY FROM LONG ILLNESS

The digestive system is most delicate immediately after illness. At first, thin oat broth may be all that can be tolerated. As the person grows stronger, try providing small amounts of well-cooked oatmeal; later, add crushed walnuts on top. Walnuts excel at rebuilding strength and promoting weight gain. Mild teas stimulate digestion — catnip, lemon balm, or dandelion — but at first, they may need to be weak infusions instead of standard strength.

Borage. Because of borage's unique building effect on the adrenal glands, it helps the body recover from stress and the lingering effects of steroid therapy, radiation, and chemotherapy. Borage seed oil, or borage leaf tea, is effective administered during and immediately after illness. As the person grows stronger, it is infinitely more fun to add fresh borage to the diet in salads, lemonades, syrups, or jams. Toss the salad with a walnut borage oil, and garnish with a few beautiful star-shaped blue borage flowers to please the eye as well as the palate.

Fresh greens. Long illness depletes the body of vital nutrients. Eat fresh greens and edible flowers to replace nutrients as efficiently as possible. Freely add alfalfa, burdock root, dandelion (flowers, greens, and roots), mallow (greens and cheeses), plantain (leaves and seeds), strawberry (leaves and blossoms), and violet (leaves and blossoms) into soups, salads, stir-fries, and desserts whenever possible, as well as strawberries, raspberries, blackberries, rose hips, and walnut meats.

Garlic. To help rebuild a weakened immune system, add 2 cloves of fresh garlic daily to the diet. Or, if the person's stomach cannot yet tolerate garlic, encourage a daily garlic footbath. Drink teas of thyme, St.-John's-wort, lemon balm, or violet to gently stimulate the immune system. St.-John's-wort and lemon balm have the additional benefit of easing the depression that invariably accompanies long-term illness.

SLEEP PROBLEMS

Catnip, lemon balm, oat straw, and rose petal teas are all mildly sedative. Blend or leave as simples according to your personal tastes.

Bedwetting at night. This can be remedied by restricting water several hours before bedtime; also, have the person take a tablespoon of honey just before retiring. The honey will absorb excess moisture and eliminate the need for frequent bathroom trips.

Oversleeping. Needing too much sleep and lethargy may be signs of depression. St.-John's-wort has been shown more effective at relieving depression than commonly prescribed pharmaceuticals, with fewer side effects. Blend it with lemon balm and borage for greater effectiveness.

Conversely, if you need to stay awake, try a cup of strong ginger tea. Its stimulating warmth will invigorate your circulatory system to give a rush of energy without leaving any caffeine jitters behind.

Insomnia. Sleep on a pillow filled with dried lavender blossom, rose petal, and catnip to ease restlessness and insomnia. Children love to make these pillows, and it is a good way to introduce them to herbalism.

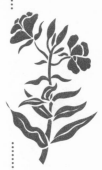

SMOKING TOBACCO (QUITTING)

Substitute herbs for tobacco. If you don't want to quit cold turkey, cut back on the amount of tobacco you use by adding herbs to it. Mullein leaf and a pinch of mint makes a fine smoke all by itself (or mullein leaf and rose petal, if you like a sweeter smoke). Each time you roll a cigarette, add more mullein and less tobacco. Most people can wean themselves from tobacco in a short time in this way.

Other herbs that make for a pleasant smoke are blackberry blossom, catnip leaf, lemon balm leaf, mullein flower, strawberry blossom, and violet flower. Old-timers used to smoke corn silk in their corncob pipes. It has a mild and pleasant taste that blends well with other herbs.

Chewing herbs. Chew on a piece of marsh mallow root or candied ginger, or on fresh rose hips.

Easing withdrawal. To ease the nervous anxiety that comes from nicotine withdrawal, use borage seed oil, and drink lemon balm or oat straw tea.

A double-blind placebo study has shown that extracts of fresh oats can reduce the craving for cigarettes. In the test, five out of the thirteen oat eaters stopped smoking, seven cut back by 50 percent, and only one person kept smoking as before. The effect lasted for as long as two months after the smokers stopped eating the oats!

Drink copious amounts of water to flush the nicotine from your body. Or take hot baths with ginger or peppermint added to bring on a sweat, cleanse the toxin from your body, and help you relax.

SORE THROATS

Nibble on fresh young borage leaf, dried or fresh mallow root, a small piece of poplar bark, or violet blossom. Or, if you are brave enough, chew a piece of fresh raw garlic for fast relief.

White pine. A strong infusion of white pine needle tea will coat the throat with its antiseptic resins and provide generous amounts of vitamins A and C. Or suck on homemade thyme and balsam poplar bud pastilles.

Herbal syrup. A teaspoon of an herbal syrup will provide relief. Syrups made from borage, catnip, garlic, lavender, lemon balm, mallow, peppermint, plantain, poplar, red clover, rose, strawberry leaf, thyme, or white pine inner bark will aid a sore throat.

Gargle. Antiseptic gargles will help combat and prevent strep throat. Make a strong tea of thyme, peppermint, garlic, or white pine inner bark; gargle and swallow.

STRAINS AND SPRAINS

Use RICE to treat strains and sprains. No, I don't mean the grain. RICE is an acronym for Rest, Ice, Compression, and Elevation. As soon as you suspect a sprain, keep the joint as motionless as possible, and elevate it over the person's head to relieve pain and swelling. Wrap it with an Ace bandage for firm support, and apply ice packs during the first twenty-four hours. Many times it's impossible to know if a hand or foot is bruised, sprained, or broken unless an x-ray is taken.

Plaintain. Plantain leaf will cool an area and provide further relief from swelling and inflammation. Bind the bruised leaves directly onto the area, wrap loosely with a compression bandage, and apply ice on top. The plantain should be changed every other hour or so. Don't leave the plantain on overnight, as it can become lumpy if the person sleeps restlessly.

After twenty-four hours, use warm compresses and soaks of herbs that help reduce swelling, bruises, and inflammation. Borage leaf, plantain, poplar bark, and violet or walnut leaf will aid the recovery process.

Tea. Drink a blend of poplar bark and lemon balm tea to ease pain and inflammation, and to lift the spirits.

MAKING A COMPRESSION BANDAGE

In some emergency situations in which a hospital is not nearby, you may need to make a field cast or compression bandage. This can be made from white pine. Put 1 pound of white pine branches, with their needles, into 1 gallon of water and boil until it is reduced by half. Strain and boil until a thin syrup forms. Dip strips of flannel or muslin into the syrup.

Now use as follows: Make sure the sprained joint is in a good position. Wrap the joint in a soft clean cloth, then follow with a layer of cotton, cattail down, or other soft filling. Finally, put on the wet cloth strips so that they form a firm but not overly tight bandage. Do **not** put the strips directly against the skin. Made properly, this bandage will lend enough support to enable the person to walk out of the wilderness with the aid of a walking stick.

WARTS

Saliva. The most convenient remedy I know of for warts is simply to rub your own saliva on them several times a day. The enzymes in your saliva that help break down the protein in your food also help break down the structure of the wart. This works very well for children, who may have a sea of warts clustered in an area. Of course, it helps to give the child a special magic chant to say when he spits on the wart. "I wish, I wish, I wish, the warts would go away." Magic and superstition, yes . . . but it always helps to believe in what you do.

Dandelion. Apply the white sap from the stem or root of dandelion directly to the wart at least once a day. It is just corrosive enough to be effective against the wart, but it leaves the surrounding tissue undamaged.

Rose hip seed oil. The high vitamin E content of rose hip seed oil will help soften stubborn plantar warts. Then dandelion juice can be applied to dissolve them away.

There are many anecdotal stories of stubborn and persistent warts disappearing when a person turns from a high-protein (meat-based) to a high-carbohydrate (vegetarian) diet.

WORMS, PARASITES, AND FUNGAL INFECTIONS

Most home remedies to expel worms and parasites incorporate modified food fasts. Eating only raw cabbage or carrots is considered a remedy by itself — but I sure can't get my children to stick to that for the three to five days required! A more successful approach is to lean the diet toward eating lots of beans, rice, cabbage, and carrots for about a week while drinking lots of water and demulcent teas (such as borage or plantain leaf), trying the herbal therapies below, and taking any side indulgences with a grain of salt.

Garlic. Garlic is superior to many prescription drugs at eliminating parasites because it often works just as fast but is much safer and less expensive to use. Garlic can wipe out *Giardia lamblia* in as little as three days, and pinworms overnight! Chop a clove of fresh garlic and take with each meal, along with one additional dose of garlic before retiring. Fresh garlic works fast and efficiently; garlic oils, capsules, and powders do not. A wash with garlic wine or garlic water as made on page 78 will quickly eliminate ringworm, athlete's foot, and other fungal infections. Since garlic's parasite-fighting qualitites are destroyed by heat, follow instructions for making simple tea from leaves and flowers on page 23. For best results, continue using the garlic until the egg-laying cycle of the parasite has passed.

Walnuts. Walnut hulls and bark expel intestinal worms and parasites from the body. They are especially useful for skin-related parasites and may be safely used both externally and internally. The one drawback is that a wash made with the hulls will stain the skin a patchy dark brown that lasts for several weeks — about as long as a Florida tan! However, since their action is sure and mild, walnuts are often employed by those who may disdain garlic for one reason or another.

PART II:
AROMATHERAPY

Creating Personal Blends
for Mind & Body

Colleen K. Dodt

CHAPTER 9
Awakening the Scent Sense

We often take our olfactory world for granted and, unless directly stimulated, ignore our sense of smell. Stop for a moment and reflect upon your personal sense of smell. Is it strong or weak? Which scents attract or repel you? Do you like floral, herbal, fruity, earthy, or spicy scents? What is your favorite scent? Your least favorite? Why do you like or dislike certain scents?

SMELL AND PERCEPTION

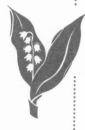

In his *Aromatherapy Workbook,* Marcel Lavabre notes that the French word *sentir* means "to smell, to feel." We "feel" scents, rather than logically think about them. There is very little language to describe scent. We understand it more through associations and images than by analytical processes or data. In the limbic portion of the brain, emotions and odors are directly linked and have been found to produce some of the same electrical impulses. The limbic system is also called the rhinencephalon, or "smell part" of the brain.

Smell plays a significant role in how we perceive places and situations. Good smells help us to feel good, bad ones depress us. Think about walking into a beautiful room, immaculate in every way. How would you feel about that room if it smelled terrible? Regardless of what you saw, the bad scent would make you uncomfortable. Likewise, imagine arriving at the door of the worst place you ever saw but, upon entering, discovering it smelled of roses. Your sense of smell would likely diminish your discomfort with the place, and make you a little more willing to explore it. Unless, of course, you have experienced a direct negative experience with the scent of roses in the past. Then your anxiety level may actually increase due to this previous scent-conditioning experience. People often associate the smell of a place such as a hospital, nursing home, or funeral home with what they experienced there. Although these places may do their best to create a clean or comfortable environment, people often have negative emotions tied to the time they spent there and to the scent they remember.

For many of us, the sense of smell is greatly diminished by sinus problems, pollution, and the synthetic aromatic chemicals we are bombarded with daily. These can reek havoc on our delicate sense of smell. I notice my sense of smell is always heightened after being closed in the steamy bathroom with aromatic essential oils. The additional heat and moisture in the air make the odor molecules more accessible to my nose. As I walk through the kitchen en route from the bathroom to the boudoir, scents in the house that usually go unnoticed suddenly come alive. The fruit bowl is redolent with ripening bananas, pears, and oranges; the coffee grinder smells of good Kona coffee; the small bottle of my personal perfume on the bedroom dresser is sweet and familiar as I search for my clothes; and when I open the towel cupboard in the bathroom, the scent of line-dried towels fills my nostrils. Is there a scent to line-dried clothes? I say yes, but I couldn't say what it is comprised of — unless sun and wind have a scent of their own.

RETRAINING YOUR SENSE OF SMELL

I have often seen clients taken aback by the scent of pure undiluted essential oils. The oils are so strong that people don't know quite how to react. Our sense of smell often requires some retraining to appreciate natural scents. These oils, which require large amounts of plant material to produce, are very concentrated!

The next time you peel an orange, squeeze a lemon, apply your favorite perfume, or stop to savor the scent of a rose, think about what you are experiencing. Write down your reaction. Be aware of your olfactory world. We are truly led by the nose! Pure essential oils make this journey a wonderful adventure.

SCENT AS PROTECTION

On a misty spring day in late March when I went out to my mailbox, I noted the scent of celery that had been left in the garden over the winter. Heat, light, air, and moisture all activate the release of scent. Smell helps orient us to place, season, and even imminent danger.

For our ancestors, the ability to find a mate, a home, or even search for food depended greatly upon olfactory acuity. Even today we detect danger with our nose. If there is a gas leak at home, the scent added to natural gas will warn us very quickly. If some leftovers in the refrigerator have been there too long, our nose will tell us not to eat them. Poisonous plants often have a bad acrid smell that warns not to ingest them, while the sweet-scented herbs that can enhance our everyday existence invite us to consume them through the release of their oils. From the day we are born, our sense of smell is an intimate link to our survival.

People who suffer anosmia, meaning they have lost their sense of smell, are often prone to depression due to the lack of scent in their world. I received a letter from a man who had worked very diligently to improve his sense of smell. He said he could smell very clearly the ink with which he was writing the letter. He asserted that if more people had an alive sense of smell instead of an often deadened one, we would not be able to tolerate the stench of the society we live in today. I couldn't help but wonder how he would have adjusted to past times of open sewage in the streets and no garbage disposal!

For a strange twist on the sense of smell, read the novel *Perfume: The Story of a Murderer,* by Patrick Suskind. In this novel set in the French countryside, life and death hinges upon a keen, obsessive olfactory sense. Another interesting account of the sense of smell is *A Natural History of The Senses,* by Diane Ackerman. Ms. Ackerman explains how the sense of smell has guided us down the dimly lit corridors of evolution. The agony of anosmia is portrayed and examined.

USING SCENT TO PRODUCE PARTICULAR RESPONSES

The subliminal use of scent to produce particular behavioral responses is widespread in our society. Scratch-and-sniff entered our children's lives long ago, and magazines aren't complete today without a scented advertisement or two. Many products contain subliminal scenting of which consumers are often totally unaware. Think about this: Do you buy a product because it cleans well or because it smells like a refreshing lemon or a pine forest? A large car manufacturer approached me once to ask if I could create "new-car" smell. I told them they needed a chemist, not an essential oil consultant. Well, they promptly found one, and they now spray "new-car" smell in their used cars to enhance sales.

Neurochemical Experiences Produced by Essential Oils

People say lavender smells clean. How can something smell clean? I know I can smell the scent of spring. I have also experienced scent in dreams. It is learned-odor responses — odors that have memories attached to them — that lead us on these olfactory emotional odysseys. Learned-odor responses arouse reactions to certain synthetic or natural scents, like the scent of an ex-lover's perfume or the smell of freshly mown grass.

However, our experience of a pure essential oil is different than a learned-odor response. When an essential oil is inhaled, various neurochemicals are released in the brain and the inhaler experiences a physiological change in body, mind, and spirit. When lavender is inhaled, for instance, serotonin is released from the raphe nucleus of the brain, producing a calming influence in the body. This effect is altered, however, if the inhaler has had a direct negative experience with lavender.

A learned-odor response can alter or interfere with the biochemical effects of essential oils. An intense emotional response to a certain odor may interfere with the chemical release from the brain. Emotions have their own chemical make-up and can be powerful enough to inhibit or enhance a neurochemical release or absorption. For this reason, over-the-counter aromatherapy formulas aren't effective for everyone, since people's life experiences are so varied. For example, if a child had a caretaker in their life who wore a certain scent such as lavender, a known relaxant, and that caretaker had a direct negative association for this particular child, it could perhaps be difficult for this person to relax when exposed to lavender because of a learned-odor response. In the same vein, an odor many find offensive, such as barnyard, may have a positive influence for one raised happily on a farm. Sweet orange essential oil has a generally uplifting association for some people.

Others find its effects sedative. However, if one has had a direct negative experience associated with this scent — such as being forced to work long and hard to harvest this fruit — you may no longer find this scent uplifting or sedative at all. This association to sweet orange would be a learned-odor response. I am not acquainted with any direct research in overcoming or changing learned-odor responses with pure essential oils.

Chemical reproductions of pure essential oils don't hold this olfactory magic and are not effective in aromatherapy. They rely solely on learned-odor response, not neurochemical release. Chemical reproductions do not have the same biochemical effects as naturally occurring pure essential oils.

The effects of essential oils are both scientific and experiential. As you become more familiar with pure essential oils and the scents that surround you in your personal worlds, the experiential influences will be greatly enhanced. I have often been comforted by a familiar scent when I was miles away from home because I associated it with the comfort of home. The neurochemical releases influence our emotional response to various essential oils and the context in which they are employed.

I have a poster produced by Tisserand Aromatherapy, Ltd., in England, entitled *Psycho-Aromatherapy,* that details the various pure essential oils and how they affect the brain. The poster quotes Edward Sagarin, who in 1945 said, "Odour is the story of language, of man's efforts to find words to express emotion and sensation. It is allied with all the senses; indissolubly with taste, with colour, sound and memory, and deeply affected by the psychological phenomenon, the power of suggestion." In small print at the bottom, it says, "The above is scientifically proven." This, to me, captures the logical, yet mysterious, way in which our sense of smell, and our experience of essential oils, influences our world.

THE HEALING EFFECTS
OF ESSENTIAL OILS

When someone walks into my house they say, "Gee, what smells so good?" It is amazing how I can see people visibly change when they come into contact with pure essential oils. Throughout history, people have believed in the healing effects of herbs. During times of plague, it was believed that the perfumers and glovers didn't fall ill because they were constantly exposed to the essential oils in their daily work. It was very fashionable to have one's gloves perfumed with pure essential oils. People also carried little nosegays or tussie mussies fashioned from freshly cut herbs and flowers. These little bouquets were held up to the nose while out in the streets in a time of, shall we say, less than adequate sanitation. The herbs and flowers, of course, contained pure essential oils. Why do you think bringing herbs and flowers to someone in the hospital started? Rosemary, thyme, and lavender herbs were burnt on hospital wards of long ago to help purify the air.

CHAPTER 10

Buying and Using
Pure Essential Oils

▼▼▼▼▼

The term "essential oil" is thrown about every day, with a wide range of meanings. There are no standardized regulations for use of the words "essential oil" or "essence," so they are often used to describe any number of products which have little or nothing to do with the real thing or meaning.

When I refer to essential oils in this book I mean the pure plant distillates and extracts that are excellent allies in yesterday's, today's, and tomorrow's world of home health care. They are naturally derived, and should be respected as powerful substances to be used with caution and education. Pure essential oils are extracted directly from different parts of plants, depending on the oil concerned. Some are extracted from flowers, others from leaves, stems, the rind of fruit, berries, resin, or roots. There are a variety of extraction methods, including distillation, expression, solvent extraction, effleurage, the phytonic process, and the super critical carbon dioxide extraction. The extraction process used depends on the plant. For example, orange, lemon, grapefruit, and bergamot are usually expressed because the oils are present in the peels and released when the peel is ruptured. Others, including lavender, clary sage, chamomile, and rose geranium, are distilled. Some flowers, like rose, are distilled

▼▼▼▼▼

WHAT IS AN ESSENTIAL OIL?

Pure essential oils are some of life's greatest pleasures. Their name itself is indicative of their status in everyday life. Webster's dictionary, which is my favorite book, defines "essential" as: 1. Of or constituting the intrinsic, fundamental nature of something; basic; inherent. 2. Absolute; complete; perfect; pure. 3. Necessary to make a thing what it is; indispensable; requisite. 4. Containing or having the properties of a concentrated extract of a plant, drug or food. Essential oils are nature by the drop, to enjoy and enhance life. They contain the life force of a valuable botanical in a form that is basic and easy to access. Anything essential is absolutely necessary, a fundamental requisite to healthier living.

▲▲▲▲▲

and solvent extracted, resulting in either a rose absolute or rose otto. The variety of rose used also makes a difference. Extraction of pure essential oils usually requires laboratory equipment and a large amount of materials for a small yield of oil. I have seen directions for homemade stills, yet found them too much bother for such a small yield. Distilling in a small ready-made still from Europe has helped me appreciate why many oils are expensive and can be difficult to locate. I, for one, will leave the extraction to those who know their business and be glad that I don't have to try to acquire my own oils by extracting them. My rosewater experience each summer is enough extraction for me, and for most home gardeners. If you are interested in trying extraction at home, you can find detailed information in books and online.

However it is extracted, the resulting oil is a highly concentrated, volatile substance that is made up of many different elements, including alcohols, esters, hydrocarbons, aldehydes, ketones, phenols, terpene alcohols, and acids. Chemists have tried to recreate essential oils in the laboratory, but, to date, they have not been 100 percent successful.

A WORD ON THE COST OF PURE ESSENTIAL OILS

I am truly grateful that there are people in the world dedicated to producing the plant material to extract pure essential oils. When I really think about how much time goes into producing the contents of one little brown bottle, I am better able to explain why they can be so costly. I, for one, am willing to pay the price of pure essential oils of the best quality.

As demand for aromatherapy-quality pure essential oils is made known, hopefully more people will realize the need to grow the material to produce them, which might make the oils more available and affordable. Sandalwood and rosewood trees are both being depleted and are in great need of being replanted. If we are to use these natural resources, we have a responsibility to replace them.

BUYING PURE ESSENTIAL OILS

As a buyer, you must beware of imitations! Better yet, be educated! Synthetic aromatic chemicals have become the norm for so long that many folks are used to them, and are unaware of the choices they have from nature's bounty. Recently, I was in a very nice little shop full of scented goodies. I approached the essential oils section and found pretty little bottles with signs and labels indicating they were filled with essential oils and aromatherapy products. The slick-looking display covered with pictures of herbs and flowers led me to believe that these were indeed the true thing, but upon closer inspection I found that all the bottles were the same price. This is a clear tip-off that you're not dealing with pure essential oils since the prices of these precious oils vary greatly, depending on their accessibility and ease of extraction. I would love to find true jasmine absolute oil at the same price as lavender oil, but I don't think that will ever happen in my lifetime! Upon smelling the sampler in this shop, my suspicions that these were synthetic aromatic chemicals, not pure essential oils, were confirmed. The shopkeeper was shocked and dismayed at my discovery. She truly thought she was offering a quality aromatherapy product, and was not properly informed by her supplier.

I have happened across this same scene time and time again around the world. The adulteration, dilution, and imitation of pure essential oils has become big business — at the consumer's expense, both financially and ethically. However, with a little education and exposure to pure essential oils, you, too, will be able to sniff out the imposters.

LOOK FOR HIGH-QUALITY OILS

The quality of even pure essential oils can vary greatly depending on the country where the plant was grown, climatic conditions, how the raw material was collected and stored, and the process used to obtain the oil. Always opt for the best quality oil available.

Know what you're looking, and smelling, for when you shop for oils. Don't be taken in by a sales pitch on the latest, greatest essential oil to hit town. Do your research and go or write to a supplier with a clear knowledge of what you want. Don't be afraid to return an oil if it is not what you wanted, or is of poor quality. I have sent many oils back and told the manufacturer I wouldn't order from them again until they showed an improvement in their quality control. Most companies are anxious to know if a bit of poor oil slipped into their inventory. This problem is most prevalent in some of the larger companies that produce great volume, or where the demand for quantities of an oil is so great that it exceeds the demand for quality.

Find Reputable Suppliers

Knowing the supplier you're buying oils from is the first step. You can shop from the suppliers listed on pages 336–338 with confidence that they are doing their best to supply only the finest, high-quality pure essential oils. Questions as to the origin and purity of an oil are usually met with enthusiasm by someone who is proud of their suppliers. However, I have had shopkeepers assure me that their oils were the best and purest, even after I knew better. So again, buyer beware.

Always look for pure essential oils packaged in full, dark glass bottles, preferably with built-in droppers. These allow you to dispense the oil one drop at a time. (Aromatherapy will, if nothing else, teach you patience!) Some oils are more viscous than others and may take a while to drop out. Some companies have adjusted the size of the dropper or bottle neck accordingly. More often than not, one must be careful. Lavender will drop out much more quickly than sandalwood or vetiver. You can also use a separate glass eyedropper, but do not store it in the bottle because the oil will eventually break down the rubber bulb at the top, which will then contaminate the oil.

Read the label carefully. Look for the term "pure essential oil" and for cautions such as, "Keep out of reach of children," and, "For external use only." These warnings are signs of a responsible company that understands the effects of their product.

Buy in Small Quantities

Whenever possible, buy small bottles. Air in unfilled bottles can accelerate the deterioration of pure essential oils. Keep the bottles cool, dark, and well-filled. I will often transfer small quantities of oils to a smaller bottle if I do not need them for a while.

Avoid Synthetic Scents

I have often wondered how we fell into using synthetics in place of pure essential oils. I believe it has a lot to do with availability. Synthetic scents can be manufactured at a standard cost and rate of production, while we have to rely upon the less-predictable graces of nature for producing pure essential oils.

I have been asked many times for peach, strawberry, apple blossom, or blueberry-scented products. In response, I ask the customer if they know of a way to extract the fragrance oil from

ESSENTIAL OIL SAFETY TIPS

◆ Buy the highest quality essential oils available to you. (I use lesser quality oils to wash my floors, but never my body.)

◆ Dispense by the drop carefully and count. Record your recipe accurately.

◆ Dilute, dilute, dilute. Very seldom is an oil used "neat" or undiluted.

◆ Use cotton swabs or cotton buds to apply pure essential oils. Using the hands and fingers may eventually contaminate the bottle. Dropper top bottles easily dispense a drop at a time, making it less likely that you will use too much essential oil or accidentally have a spill.

◆ Be careful where you set your essential oil bottles and wipe them clean first. Essential oils can mar surfaces, especially plastic ones. Always make sure bottle caps are twisted on securely.

◆ Practice aromatic etiquette. Many scents may be perceived as offensive to others. Use essential oils and perfumes in moderation in public, and check with family members to make sure your precious vapors aren't causing anyone else distress because of allergies, asthma, or just personal preference.

◆ Label everything — for your own convenience and others' safety. Clearly label and put up away from children any potentially harmful substances. Labeling is a great chance to be creative, too.

these plants. When they reply "no," I assure them that no one else has either, and explain the difference between pure essential oils and synthetic aromatic chemicals.

If you like a certain synthetic scent, fine; use it to scent carpet or to perfume a room spray. Just keep in mind that pure essential oils have qualities and benefits that go beyond the scent. Peach potpourri with aqua-colored wood chips doesn't hold the same magic as a sachet of freshly dried lavender, mint, and rosemary. When squeezed, this sachet releases the pure essential oils from the tiny holding cells in the leaves and flowers. Deeply inhaling synthetic peach potpourri is just not the same and doesn't have the same benefits as inhaling the sweet, deep essential scents of lavender, mint, and rosemary.

I've found from selling my own products at the local farmer's market that consumers are often confused about what they are buying because they've seen so many synthetic concoctions. For instance, my small bottles of freshly made body oils — to which I often add a few herbs or flower buds as well as essential oils — resemble the bottled oils sold just for decoration. Many of those contain artificial, dyed, or decayed flowers and questionable base oils. Their quality doesn't compare to the pure ones I make myself. I must often remind clients that the oils I make are meant to be used, not just admired. It's all part of the educational process.

PRECAUTIONS AND CAUTIONS

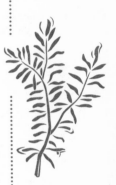

Working with pure essential oils can be rewarding in many ways. However, it can also be dangerous if certain precautions and cautions aren't observed. Remember that everyone is different and will react to individual essential oils in varying manners. The following simple precautions can make your experiences much more pleasant.

Keep Away from Eyes

Never use essential oils too near the eyes. Keep your hands away from the face, genitals, and mucous membranes when they have been in contact with oils. Always wash your hands before and after working with oils. I wear eye protection when pouring essential oils, and recommend it for you as well. If you do get some oil in the eye, wipe it with a cotton bud that has been moistened with sweet almond oil. Water will just disperse and spread the oil.

Keep Out of the Reach of Children

Pure essential oils can be toxic if ingested in large amounts, and harmful to the skin and eyes if improperly spilled or undiluted.

Children have no place playing with oils unless properly supervised and cautioned.

The use of essential oils on babies is debatable. Some sources say yes, some no. I would not use them on an infant without proper supervision and direction, such as reading *Aromatherapy for Pregnancy and Childbirth* by Margaret Fawcett, attending classes or workshops on the subject, or by visiting a qualified aromatherapist or doctor with experience in this area. I have seen success with using oils on children as young as two years old, and have successfully employed them with my own daughter, Christina, over the years. Lightly scented baths often helped her unwind, right up to today, her first in high school. Evening foot massages have proven relaxing for her many a night.

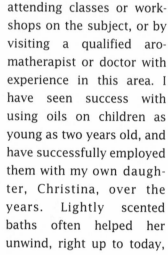

BEWARE OF MEDICINAL CLAIMS

I always advise CAUTION regarding healing and medicinal claims made by some when referring to the powers of pure essential oils. ALWAYS consult qualified help when deciding whether to use oils for something other than simple home use. Be sure to consult your doctor before changing any medications or healing practices.

Children's reactions to pure essential oils vary greatly. Christina had strong positive or negative feelings about oils and strong scents in general. Children, just like adults, take time to adjust to new things including new scents. Let their noses be their guides. Ask them which scents they like and why. The olfactory anchors you create today can span a lifetime.

Practice Caution During Pregnancy

There are conflicting opinions on the uses of essential oils during pregnancy. I have heard that absolutely no essential oils should be used in pregnancy, but I also have books detailing just how much you can use. I would advise extreme caution, especially in the first trimester. Many oils can stimulate the uterus, which may be great as birth approaches, but not at two months into the pregnancy.

I have attended births where pure essential oils were used along with jasmine absolute with marvelous results. If you are interested in this use, I advise working with a doctor, midwife, or aromatherapist who specializes in this area. I have heard reports of a reduction in stretch marks when a combination of pure essential oils and very high-quality carrier oils were used faithfully on the skin after the first trimester.

For External Use Only

Pure essential oils are meant for external use only. There are those who practice internal use, but they are doctors or professionals trained in the practice of Medicinal Aromatherapy, primarily in Europe. Using pure essential oils internally would require a great amount of training and testing before it became acceptable in America. I do not suggest that anyone use them internally for any reason.

Avoid Sun Exposure

Some essential oils, including bergamot and other citrus oils, such as lemon and orange, may increase the skin's sensitivity to the sun. The citrus oils can also increase the skin pigmentation in some people. If not properly blended and applied unevenly, darkening and skin irritation could result. According to *Principals of Holistic Skin Therapy With Herbal Essences,* by Dietrich Gumbel, the skin generally has a good reception to citrus oils when properly diluted, applied, and not exposed to direct sunlight. You can

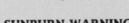

SUNBURN WARNING

Avoid exposing skin to direct sunlight within six hours of applying citrus oils such as bergamot, lemon, and orange oils. These oils contain components that may cause reddening and blistering or darkening of the skin when exposed to sunlight.

purchase bergamot with the bergaptene (the component of the oil that can lead to increased pigmentation of the skin) removed.

Lemongrass, a fast-growing grass often used in culinary arts, and spice oils such as cinnamon and clove have an irritant effect when used directly upon the skin, due to some of the key chemical constitutes they contain. I saw one client who had a very strong reaction to too much lemongrass (4 ml) she added to a bath. Her skin became red and inflamed, causing her a lot of discomfort. This was alleviated by washing well with soap, showering, and treating her skin with soothing oil mixed with a small amount of lavender, and Roman chamomile.

Remember the Oils Are Concentrated

Pure essential oils and absolutes are very concentrated. Many pounds of herbs, flowers, resins, or fruits are used to produce small amounts of oils. Only small amounts of oil are needed to gain results. "Less is best" is what I tell my work-study students and clients. Many people think that if two drops of an oil will help them feel better, than five or six drops will lead to greater relaxation or stimulation — not so! Using too much essential oil can sometimes have a boomerang effect and aggravate, rather than soothe, symptoms. Essential oils can be expensive, and using less is smart in a financial sense as well.

Use Them Diluted

Pure essential oils are almost always used in dilution. Very seldom are they used "neat," meaning undiluted, or straight. Lavender is one oil I feel confident using neat. Tea tree, sandalwood, patchouli, jasmine, and rose absolute have never given me a problem neat. I dab sweet lavender neat on small cuts, scrapes, burns, bumps, and insect bites.

Most other essential oils I use in a dilution of sweet almond oil (see page 174 for exact proportions) or some other base or carrier oil such as grapeseed, apricot kernel, or jojoba (which is actually a liquid wax). For a less oily blend, you can add the oils to a high-quality, unscented cream or lotion base.

Essential oils can also be diluted into shampoos, hair rinses, spring water, alcohol, gels, lotions, and creams. When added to shampoos and rinses, the oils enhance the natural beauty of hair. When added to alcohol, they become elegant perfumes. Another application method is to dilute the oil in a bowl of warm water and use with a compress, or dilute it in a carrier oil or cream that can then be used to massage or condition the skin. Some people suggest diluting oils in milk or cream before adding to a bath, but I just add them directly to the water and stir well. Some people actually prefer the smell of diluted essential oils over the intense smell of the concentrated oil.

Beware of Heat Sources

Keep a keen eye on any heat source you employ to release the scent of essential oils. Candles, simmer pots, and light-bulb rings can catch fire if not properly attended. Forgo using these methods when you are ill or very sleepy. A diffuser on a timer will serve you much better — and keep you safer. Oils on cotton or a small cloth work well when you're tired as well.

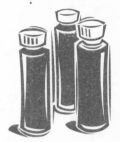

CHAPTER 11

Properties and Applications
of Essential Oils

▼▼▼▼

The application of pure essential oils in your life can bring about significant benefit and change when properly employed. Researchers in Europe and America have been studying these precious substances for many years. Long before the term aromatherapy became popular, doctors in France were using essential oils to treat those wounded in wars when medical supplies ran short. Dr. Jean Valnet, M.D., addresses the medicinal uses as well as the antiseptic powers of pure essential oils in his book, *The Practice of Aromatherapy, Holistic Health and the Essential Oils of Flowers and Herbs*. I encourage you to take the time to research the individual essential oils you want to incorporate into your life on your own, as well as checking references by those who have found success in their use. There are several aromatherapy journals available that detail case histories and research. Most are from England, and well worth the price of a subscription. The people submitting these findings have first-hand knowledge and their personal experiences are invaluable to those just beginning their aromatic endeavors.

MOST COMMONLY USED
PURE ESSENTIAL OILS

The following pure essential oils are the ones I tend to use the most. They are also ones I have found my clients and customers seem to use and ask for often. This list is only a sampler of essential oils, absolutes, and oleoresins that are available. Most are usually easy to obtain and aren't too cost prohibitive to use. Rose and jasmine are expensive, but are usually used in diluted form and purchased in small amounts. If you have a friend who is also interested in using essential oils, you might go in together to buy a bottle of an essence or absolute that is cost-prohibitive to buy on your own. All of the following essential oils have a broad variety of uses, and most blend together quite well.

BERGAMOT *(Citrus bergamia)*

Nature: The scent of bergamot is delightful, fresh, uplifting, and clean. It stands on its own, or blends well with most other oils. To me, it is a citrus/floral scent. This is a nice addition to personal scents for both men and women.

Benefits: Bergamot is balancing, regenerating, and a necessary essential in every household. This oil seems to have the power to help lift melancholia and depression.

Suggested Uses/Blending: I personally blend this oil with patchouli, lavender, and rose absolute for an all-purpose blend that I use on every inch of my body. I dab this blend neat on little spots or bumps. I also like to blend it with sea salt and bathe in it.

Caution: Exposure to the sun can result in a darkening of the skin to which this oil has been applied. I put this to the test a few summers ago by applying neat bergamot on my thumb while I was gardening. Sure enough, that thumb got much darker than the rest of my hand. The darkening of the pigmentation lasted well into the next spring! It was strange being a gardener with a brown thumb. It reminded me of the time I burned my hand badly with a hot glue gun and treated just part of the burn with lavender and vitamin E — once healed, this area didn't even have a scar.

These kinds of experiments have thoroughly convinced me of the healing powers of pure essential oils. Try your own experiments and you'll see what I mean.

CLARY SAGE *(Salvia sclarea)*

Nature: Clary sage is a most interesting essential oil. It has become an important part of many of my blends and a favorite herb in the garden. The whorls of flowers are so perfect and beautiful that it seems perfect that they produce a unique essential oil. I love to pass clary sage in the garden, my skirt often rubbing against the leaves and absorbing the oils, only to have them waft up to me later as I sit in the sun.

Benefits: Clary sage has been found to be anti-depressant, anti-anxiety, uplifting, antispasmodic, anti-inflammatory, aphrodisiac, an aid to deeper sleep, and a benefit to the skin and hair.

Suggested Uses: Clary sage has a place in many body-care products, especially those for hair and skin. I favor it in a hair oil and as a relaxing, regulating addition to shampoos and conditioners. Its antidepressant properties provide an extra bonus in my beauty routine.

As a woman, I would not be without clary sage oil. Its distinct scent has helped me through premenstrual days with grace and ease, as it will through menopause, as well.

Clary sage is effective for men also, and I have known men who love its interesting aroma.

Caution: Some caution must be observed with dear clary as she can get quite out of hand if used too often in too high a dilution. There have been reports of intoxication with clary sage and it is advised never to mix its use with the consumption of alcoholic beverages. Clary is also best avoided in the first months of pregnancy. Use caution when driving after exposure to clary sage. I reserve it for those relaxing times when I can simply rest after its use.

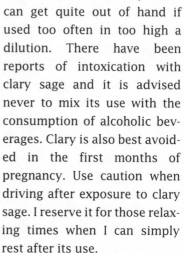

SUGGESTED RECIPES FOR CLARY SAGE

To enhance shampoo or conditioner: Add 1 to 2 drops to ½ ounce of shampoo or conditioner.

For premenstrual symptoms: Blend 3 to 6 drops with 1 to 2 drops of rose otto and 3 to 5 drops of lavender and add to a tub full of warm bathwater.

EUCALYPTUS (*Eucalyptus globulus*)

Nature: Eucalyptus is probably the best-known pure essential oil. Its clean, healing scent reminds many people of some type of medicine. I am often told this oil smells like Vicks VapoRub, a popular chest rub salve. I reply, "No, Vicks smells like eucalyptus." There are many types of eucalyptus, including a lemon one, *Eucalyptus citriodora*.

Benefits: Eucalyptus is an effective insect repellant, and can benefit the skin by acting as an antidote to bites and stings. It also has been found to help relieve neuralgia and muscular aches and pains. I have included eucalyptus in antirheumatic massage oils and chest rubs.

Eucalyptus is believed to be balancing, antiseptic, antidiabetic, antiviral, decongestant, expectorant, insect repellant, fever-reducing, and disinfectant. It has been found effective in cases of asthma. (**Caution:** Some asthma is triggered by strong odors.) **Suggested Uses:** Eucalyptus has a place in every household. Its antiseptic properties have made it a staple in cases of infectious diseases and epidemics. Its opening powers make it invaluable in fighting sinus and chest congestion. I always burn it in a simmer pot when there is illness in the house to protect anyone who stops by, and to purify and clear the air.

Eucalyptus is a very important ingredient in my world-famous, super-duper, extra-powerful Sniffy Bag™. These little bags were first blended for my daughter when she was quite young and had a bit of a running nose or congestion. She was a breast-fed child, so I would slip the bag into my blouse so she could inhale and nurse comfortably. At night, I would slip one into her pillow and she would wake clear and refreshed.

The Sniffy Bag™ lasts indefinitely if stored in a glass jar when not in use. It can always be rejuvenated with the blend of pure essential oils that are part of its contents which are, of course, called Sniffy Oil™. This oil is a must in cough, cold, congestion, and bronchial remedies. It may, however, antidote homeopathic remedies so you should choose one type of treatment or the

MAKE YOUR OWN SNIFFY BAG AND OIL

You can create your own sniffy bag by combining equal parts of crushed eucalyptus, peppermint, coltsfoot, and comfrey herbs. The peppermint, coltsfoot, and comfrey are easily grown in a household garden. The eucalyptus can be obtained from a health food store or herb supplier. If you live in a year-round warm climate, you may be able to grow the eucalyptus. I saw lovely large trees while touring herb businesses in California.

To make your own sniffy oil to add to the sniffy bag, combine five parts eucalyptus oil to one part peppermint oil. Combine the sniffy bag herbs first, then add the oil, and mix thoroughly. Put approximately ½ ounce of this mixture in a clean old sock, knot the end, place it to the nose, and inhale. To store your sniffy bag, place it in a glass, airtight jar to keep the volatile essential oils intact. If you forget to seal it in a jar, simply pour the sniffy bag contents into a bowl, add 8 to 10 drops of sniffy oil, and return it to a new clean odd sock or a small cloth bag.

For a sniffy bath, add 6 to 8 drops of sniffy oil blend directly to the bathwater, or toss in a sniffy bag. This is great to do whenever you feel a cold coming on.

other. This has always been a dilemma for me; I must consider each case individually to discern which is most needed. Store eucalyptus well away from any homeopathic remedies.

GRAPEFRUIT *(Citris paradisi)*

Nature: Grapefruit is bright, uplifting, clean, and euphoric. It is also cleansing, clearing, and stimulating to the lymphatic system.

Benefits: Grapefruit is believed to help balance the appetite, and has been found useful in treating obesity. It has also been effective in helping to balance the emotions, and has gained high marks from aromatherapists in aiding mood swings. I have personally found it to be very valuable in lifting my spirits. During times of emotional imbalance, grapefruit was there to aid me when all the medical community offered was prescription drugs which weren't the answer for me. Along with juniper, grapefruit is toning to the skin. It is believed to help rid the body of cellulite by cleansing away toxins. It has also been found useful in relieving water retention, congested skin, nervous exhaustion, and stress.

Suggested Uses: I employ grapefruit in baths, massage oils, and skin care. It is the ingredient in my "skinny bath," (see recipe on page 139). The scent is so fresh that I often use it to start a gray, cloudy day when it's often hard to get up and carry on. It seems impossible to stay depressed any length of time with sunny grapefruit as an ally. It is a wonderful citrus note in a personal essence, and I like to put a citrine stone in the bottle to mix it.

Blending: Grapefruit blends well with most oils and adds that light, refreshing note found in summer colognes.

SUGGESTED RECIPES FOR GRAPEFRUIT OIL

For uplifting the spirits: Place a cloth with a few drops of grapefruit oil on the warm clothes dryer in the basement or laundry room and let its uplifting essence waft throughout the house.

For jet lag: Blend 10 drops each of grapefruit, bergamot, and lavender oils in 1 dram (4 ml) of base oil. Rub it into the hands and inhale as needed. Or, add 2 drops of each of the above-mentioned oils undiluted or neat to a bath. I found this blend highly effective in lifting my mood when I arrived in England exhausted from many hours of travel and while trying to adjust to different time zones.

JASMINE ABSOLUTE (*Jasminum officinale*)

Nature: Jasmine, sweet jasmine is one scent nearly everyone loves. It is deep, sweet, floral, and rich. Real jasmine, like rose, is beyond comparison to the imitation fragrances that fill shop shelves.

Benefits: Jasmine is believed to be antidepressant, warming, anti-anxiety, beneficial to the skin and scalp, aphrodisiac, emotionally balancing, soothing, antiseptic, and sedative. Jasmine absolute has been found effective in cases of impotence, frigidity, lethargy, fear, and lack of confidence.

Suggested Uses: A few drops of true jasmine add a heady richness to a personal essence. Added to skin-care products and hair oils, it helps to soothe and moisturize. I love to apply jasmine in my hair and inhale its precious vapors all day long. I apply it by spreading a drop of the pure undiluted absolute across my fingertips and lacing my hair just after washing. A drop of sandalwood is nice as well. This is a wonderful personal treat, especially when I'm on my way to appointments where confidence and emotional balance are a priority. The scent seems to help me feel more beautiful and ready to face the day. One added bonus is having complete strangers approach you in public and comment on how wonderful your perfume is.

> ### SUGGESTED RECIPE FOR JASMINE ABSOLUTE
>
> **For hair care:** Combine 2 drops jasmine, 30 drops rosemary, 10 drops lavender, 5 drops clary sage, 3 drops patchouli, and 5 drops sandalwood in a 4-ml amber bottle (label it "Hair Care"). Carry it in your purse and lace 3 drops through your hair with your fingertips, or 3 drops on your hair brush and brush through your hair, as needed, to refresh yourself.

Long considered an aphrodisiac, jasmine is an important ingredient in my Love Oil. It is uplifting, and seems to exude confidence. Blended with patchouli, rose, sandalwood, and ylang-ylang, jasmine brings out sensuality. It is used in treating impotence and frigidity with great success, because it relaxes the body and soothes the emotions.

Jasmine is the oil of choice for massaging a mother about to give birth, but is too stimulating to be used in early pregnancy. Jasmine massage oil makes a wonderful baby shower gift. It can be very costly, but, like rose, well worth the expense.

To combat depression, try wearing jasmine as a personal essence and let it envelope you throughout the day in a fragrance that has been cherished for centuries by many cultures. Just breathing in the jasmine essence is believed to benefit the respiratory system. Jasmine is a very important part of my personal essence, CKD I (see page 185).

Blending: I dilute jasmine in jojoba oil before use, a blend that keeps longer than one made with sweet almond oil. Only a very small amount of jasmine is needed — do not be tempted to use more for a greater effect, since it may actually have an opposite effect when used in too high a dilution. Less is best. Besides, the cost of good true jasmine will limit its use for most folks.

JUNIPER *(Juniperus communis)*

Nature: Juniper has been a favorite of mine for many years. Its scent seems sacred to me and always clears my mind. I like to add a few drops each of juniper and frankincense to self-igniting charcoal blocks to burn as incense. (**Caution:** Place on a fire- or heat-proof surface. The blocks get glowing red.)

Benefits: I associate the scent of juniper with improved overall health. It is believed to be antiseptic, astringent, diuretic, cleansing, detoxifying, tonic, antispasmodic, parasiticidal, and antirheumatic. Juniper oil has been found useful in cases of edema, skin care, emotional imbalance, diabetes, arthritis, and cleaning.

Juniper has been said to help relieve cellulitis by detoxifying and enabling the body to throw off toxic wastes that accumulate as a result of our contemporary lifestyle. It aids in opening and cleansing the skin, thus enabling it to function more efficiently at eliminating toxins.

Suggested Uses: Juniper is useful in skin-care preparations. It makes an excellent addition to a hair oil, and is wonderful when combined with rosemary and jasmine.

My favorite way to use juniper is in what I call my "skinny bath" (see recipe). Before bathing, I do a salt glow (see recipe on pages 166–167). This helps to eliminate toxins in the body and has helped me shed a few unwanted pounds in short order. Use caution, though, to make sure that the oils and water in your bath are well mixed. I once jumped out of the tub too quickly and some neat juniper oil clung to my hip. The result was an inflamed spot that needed immediate attention. I follow my "skinny bath" up with a massage oil of juniper, grapefruit, and cypress blended in sweet almond oil (see recipe). I like to do these treatments before retiring for the night or as a morning wake-up call, since they can be either relaxing or stimulating, depending upon my state of mind and physical condition.

Juniper has been respected as an antiseptic for centuries. It was employed to clean and disinfect castle and cottage alike. When added to cleaning water, it purifies a home and leaves a clean, woodsy scent. It can be spiritually cleansing as well, and an aid in times when emotions are drained and in need of support.

Juniper also can be used to help rid pets of unwanted vermin, as well as improve their skin.

Caution: Juniper oil should not be used in the first two trimesters of pregnancy or by those who have kidney problems since it may prove too stimulating.

SUGGESTED RECIPES FOR JUNIPER OIL

For a "skinny bath": Add 5 drops juniper oil and 3 drops grapefruit oil to a warm bath.

For "skinny massage oil": Blend 8 drops juniper oil, 5 drops grapefruit oil, and 5 drops cypress oil in a base of 2 ounces sweet almond oil, or an unscented cream or lotion. Add 2 drops of geranium, lavender, and/or rosemary oils, if desired.

For soothing arthritic limbs: Blend 5 drops juniper oil, 5 drops rosemary oil, 5 drops eucalyptus oil, and 5 drops lavender oil in 2 ounces of sweet almond oil, or your favorite base.

For improving a pet's skin: Add 4 drops directly to bathwater, or blend 2 drops juniper with 2 drops of lavender and mix well into ½ cup powder base (see page 172) to sprinkle on pet as a preventive powder. Another effective formula is 5 drops juniper and 10 drops lavender blended in an 8-ounce spritz bottle of water and used to spray a pet's sleeping quarters or areas they frequent in the home. Add 2 drops of eucalyptus to the spray to help freshen pet's quarters and deter unwanted little guests that may bug your pet.

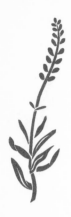

LAVENDER *(Lavandula officinalis)*

Nature: Lavender's classic floral/herbal scent has been treasured for centuries as a washing herb, and has freshened many a bed linen. Its name evolved from the Latin *lavare,* which means "to wash."

Lavender pure essential oil comes from a number of types of lavender. Its quality and scent may vary — from ones that I think smell like floor wash to ones that smell like heaven. My favorite lavender oil was a small bottle that came through a friend from the Apt region of France. It was wild lavender, or lavender savage, and I truly loved the scent. I still open the bottle years later just to savor the lingering scent.

Benefits: Lavender has been found to be antifungal, antiseptic, antidepressant, calming, normalizing, harmonizing, deodorizing, rejuvenating, anti-inflammatory, anti-bacterial, and is believed to enhance the immune system.

Lavender essential oil has been found effective in cases of stress, insomnia, acne, infection, anxiety, depression, headaches, skin irritations (burns, eczema), and fatigue.

Suggested Uses: Lavender essential oil is what I refer to as my "desert island" oil. It is the one pure essential oil that I am *never* without if I can help it! I have used it when no other was available, and found new uses for it often by trial and error. I have eased busy days into tranquil nights by adding just a drop or two of lavender oil to a tissue, or by packaging the tiny lavender flower buds inside a sachet that can be softly squeezed to release its aromatic oil. I've passed many a summer afternoon making lavender wands. These are stalks of fresh lavender flowers woven with thin satin ribbon into little wands that can be tucked into drawers or luggage.

In the garden, lavender always has a stately green/gray presence. Its flowers, when picked before they open, retain their essence for many years. In my home, I have come across some lavender flowers that have been here for a very long time. Though they are bleached of most of their lovely purple hue, they still smell sweet when crushed. I often just put a handful of lavender buds into a favorite clean odd sock, knot it up, and toss it into a linen drawer. Then I give the sock a squeeze each time I reach in to get a towel, sheet, or washcloth. Lovely lavender smells the same even if devoid of lace, and surely keeps the moths at bay in a much kinder manner than mothballs.

I have often heard stories of memories stirred by the scent of lavender and their association to a loved one. Although the scent of mothballs may conjure up a learned-odor response, the effect is not nearly so sweet, nor nearly so loved, as that of lavender.

Lavender is an essential oil that I count on for small scrapes and insect stings. It is one of the few oils that I feel safe using "neat," or undiluted on my skin. It is a favorite when a blemish pops up at just the wrong time. I simply put a drop on a cotton swab and apply it to the spot. It is very useful in skin care because of its cytophylactic, or cell-protecting and regenerating properties. I have used it successfully on burns received from glue guns or cooking on my woodstove. I keep little bottles on hand during my herb wreath classes in case anyone has a run-in with a blob of hot melted glue.

I often use lavender when traveling on planes to clear the air. However, I knew I had overdone it on a flight to California once when a gentleman seated behind me turned to his wife and asked her if she smelled bug spray! I'm not sure where he got that association, but for me the lavender scent helped me stay relaxed and made the flight much more pleasant.

Blending: Lavender blends with many other essential oils for enhanced healing properties. Some people in France actually use lavender as a base oil. I like to blend lavender with

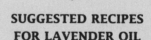

SUGGESTED RECIPES FOR LAVENDER OIL

For sunburn relief: 10 drops of lavender oil combined with 4 ounces of water in a spray bottle.

For a peaceful night's sleep: 6 to 8 drops in a simmer pot next to the bed. Be sure to keep an eye on the water level. An aromatic diffuser would also work well for dispensing the oil into the room.

For anxiety or depression: 3 to 5 drops on a tissue you carry with you.

For fresh clothes: Several drops added to the final rinse of the washer, or several drops on a cloth tossed in with the dryer load.

For more enjoyable, refreshing housecleaning: 10 to 20 drops added to 1 gallon (4 litres) of cleaning water to use around the house.

rosewood, bergamot, ylang-ylang, and lemon. It also blends well with rose and jasmine absolute, or sandalwood for an exotic perfume.

LEMON *(Citrus limonum)*

Nature: Lemon is a fragrance recognized and loved everywhere. It is a bright, sunny ally to the body, mind, and spirit. The yellow rind yields an essential oil that has numerous uses. Lemon is mentioned consistently through herbal and aromatherapy teachings for toning the skin and helping to balance oily skin. Its use is ancient and far-reaching.

Benefits: Lemon has been found to be antiseptic, astringent, bacteriostatic, and rejuvenating. The essential oil has been found effective in cases of varicose veins, gastric ulcers, skin care, depression, anxiety, and digestive problems.

Suggested Uses: Lemon is great at the start of a meal or a new day. When dining away from home, I always ask for lemon and water. I squeeze the lemon wedge into my water and savor the oil by rubbing my hands together and inhaling the pungent brightness that is lemon. Lemon juice in hot water and a dash of freshly grated ginger root eases the stomach and the sniffles.

CAUTION

The pure essential oil of lemon is much more concentrated than lemon juice, and must be treated with caution and diluted properly before applied to the skin.

As with all citrus oils, avoid direct sun exposure for up to six hours after applying essential oil of lemon on the skin.

Lemon is essential in the home. A sinkful of dishes is made much pleasanter to wash when six to eight drops of lemon essential oil are added to the water — and your hands benefit as much as your nose. Being a gardener, I appreciate the bleaching action of lemon on my nails. Doing the dishes after a day of tending my precious plants is not so bad with uplifting lemon. Once you've squeezed lemons for juice, throw the rinds into a dishpan of sudsy water and use to cut the grease on dishes. I see from the ingredient list on many hand cleaners in auto stores that manufacturers have figured out how well astringent lemon cleans, as well.

I use lemon juice to cleanse small cuts. It stings, but its healing properties are worth a bit of initial discomfort. (Lemon has been found to stimulate the production of white blood cells and aid the body in defense against infections.) Lemon is great for an uplifting bath or massage when properly diluted. The juice and pure essential oils make good hair rinses, especially for blonds. I often wonder how we've come to use synthetic lemon products when fresh lemon is so available and safe to use.

ORANGE, SWEET *(Citrus aurantium)*

Nature: Sweet orange is a tangy, sunny, bright, uplifting, refreshing scent.

Benefits: Uplifting, skin care, regenerative, antispasmodic, balancing and sedative for some. Sweet orange is an important ingredient in my Uplifting Blend (see recipe).

Suggested Uses: Sweet orange oil is inexpensive and can be used lavishly, if one so chooses. I use it around the house to clean and lighten up the environment. I have also found that a combination of sweet orange, borax, and lavender is an effective carpet treatment for deterring insects, especially fleas.

Children love the scent of fresh, fragrant orange. It is as though someone is sitting next to you, peeling this sweet fruit. Mixed with water, it makes a deodorizing room spray that is effective in dispelling melancholy or depression. A drop or two, no more, is wonderful when combined with vanilla in a bath for children.

SUGGESTED RECIPE FOR SWEET ORANGE

As an Uplifting Blend: Combine 20 drops sweet orange, 20 drops lavender, 10 drops grapefruit, 5 drops lime, 5 drops rosemary, and 2 drops jasmine absolute in a 4-ml amber bottle. Spread 3 to 5 drops across your fingertips and lace through your hair. Or add 2 drops to a tissue and inhale, or add 8 drops to a bath. 15 drops blended into 2 ounces of base can enhance a massage and revive a weary spirit. Try adding a few drops of this blend to cleaning water when a task seems particularly daunting.

I reserve this blend for times when life seems to be getting me down and I don't have time to indulge in self-pity. The scent is refreshing and stimulating. Some clients report it relaxes them quite nicely, but I prefer neroli (an essence from the orange flower) for relaxation.

Caution: Use caution when exposing skin to sun after oil is applied; some orange oil can make the skin photosensitive. Never leave children to use pure essential oils on their own. They get overly enthusiastic and always use too much! Less is always best when using pure essential oils.

PATCHOULI *(Pogostemon patchouli)*

Nature: Patchouli is not a middle-of-the-road essential oil. It evokes very strong emotional reactions from both men and women. Many associate the scent with that of moist earth, or memories of the hippie generation of the 1960s. Patchouli has enjoyed a history of being considered aphrodisiac.

Traditionally, the scent of patchouli was associated with handmade Indian shawls, which were packed in the leaves of patchouli to ward off insects. My Earth's Essence™ potpourri (see recipe on page 151), which I have made for more than ten years, is a blend of patchouli, sandalwood, and the essential oils and herbs like lavender that have been associated with protecting clothes and linens.

Benefits: Patchouli is deep and tenuous. Its scent lingers long after other essential oils have faded. It is a good base note in a personal perfume when used sparingly. Patchouli is probably the most abused essential oil when it comes to overuse. Very little is needed to create a long-lasting, lovely, personal essence, massage oil, or skin-care blend. Patchouli adds a depth to blends, and always helps me come down to earth.

Patchouli is believed to be anti-depressant, anti-inflammatory, antiseptic, deodorant, sedative in low doses, and stimulating in high doses. It is also used as a fungicide, cytophylactic, aphrodisiac, and an aid for dry cracked skin conditions.

SUGGESTED RECIPE FOR PATCHOULI

As a fortifying blend: Combine 10 drops lavender, 10 drops bergamot, 5 drops patchouli, 2 drops rose absolute in a 4 ml bottle (amounts may be doubled to fill the bottle). Add blend to a bath, or combine a drop of the blend with a few drops of water in your palm and lace through the hair, or apply under arms or behind knees to quickly brighten the senses and revive the spirits. Try altering the proportions according to taste.

Suggested Uses: Use patchouli in hair-care blends; personal essences where a deep, earthy note is desired; and baths that are heady, sensuous, and good for the skin.

PEPPERMINT *(Mentha x piperita)*

Nature: Peppermint is a favorite of many people. This herb has touched the masses through flavored breath mints, toothpaste, and sore muscle liniments.

Peppermint is piercing and pungent. Its aromatic coolness is felt as much as smelled. At times, it seems so cold that it is warming, and always must be properly diluted before use. Peppermint oil is strong, sharp, and intrusive, just like its herbal namesake in the garden.

Benefits: Peppermint has been found to be uplifting, rejuvenating, clearing, refreshing, antiseptic, an expectorant, and a mental stimulant. It is also believed to be antiseptic and antispasmodic. The essential oil has been found effective in cases of headaches, congestion, fever, fatigue, sinus headache, migraine, and muscle soreness.

Suggested Uses: Peppermint's cooling effects are appreciated after a day's work outside in the heat. After a peppermint bath you'll feel refreshed and cooler. After emerging from the bath, I like to lie down, put a small fan on low, and fall asleep before the humid weather melts my peppermint aura. My daughter always enjoyed one of these baths when she would come in dusty from a day's play and too tired to fall asleep. Peppermint is too stimulating, however, for a late-night bath. Remember, less is best — you never need much peppermint oil to do a cool job. I often use the fresh or dried herb in place of the oil when only a small amount of essence is needed.

> ### SUGGESTED RECIPES FOR PEPPERMINT
>
> **For a cool, refreshing bath:** Add 2 to 4 drops of oil to a tub full of water (do not exceed this amount!).
>
> **To relieve congestion:** Blend 1 drop peppermint, 2 drops eucalyptus, and 1 drop frankincense with ½ gallon (2 liters) of warm water in a sink or large bowl. Cover the head with a towel, hold over the mixture, relax, and breath deeply.
>
> **For sore, overworked muscles:** Prepare a massage oil of a base oil with 1 percent peppermint and 1 percent lavender. This is helpful for massaging into the body when you feel a cold or aches of flu coming on.

Peppermint tea from the fresh or dried herb has been used for centuries to settle the stomach.

Blending: Peppermint oil is blended with other oils to help relieve congestion, and it is also used as an inhalation in warm water.

Caution: Peppermint is believed to cancel the effectiveness of some homeopathic remedies, as does eucalyptus. I recommend using either the homeopathic remedies or the peppermint and eucalyptus. Always store homeopathic remedies separately from pure essential oils.

ROSE *(Rosa gallica), (Rosa damascena), (Rosa centifolia)*

Nature: Once you have inhaled the heavenly scent of rose otto or absolute, you will never again accept an imitation rose fragrance! As I write this, my roses are just coming into bud, awaiting distillation. This is my favorite time of the year, when the whole yard smells of roses, valerian in full flower, and freshly mown grass.

Benefits: Rose is believed to be an antidepressant, antiseptic, sedative, aphrodisiac, tonic, astringent, and antispasmodic. The oil has been found effective in cases of depression, insomnia, impotence, skin care, nervous tension, feminine complaints, grief, sadness, and low self-esteem.

Rose otto is produced through distillation of the flowers. I don't have enough roses to produce the oil, so I usually opt for producing a high-quality rosewater. This is obtained by distilling roses in a small still, which yields about 32 ounces of pure rosewater. When I am distilling, I'm told that the scent even reaches out to my neighbors several houses away! I wish more people could be exposed to this fragrant process. I don't recommend most of the commercial products labeled rosewater, since they usually contain a synthetic rose fragrance, not true rose oil. You can try making your own rosewater blend by adding two drops rose otto to four ounces spring water. Keep refrigerated because this contains no preservatives.

I do keep the actual rose otto on hand for very special blends that need a bit of extra love. Rose otto oil is solid when cool and warms up to a liquid in seconds when held in the hand. It is expensive and worth every cent you spend.

Suggested Uses: Rosewater has been employed as a skin-care agent for centuries. Almost all of my roses go into the production of this precious liquid, and I am very stingy with it. I like to make it last throughout the year. To do this, try storing rosewater in the refrigerator in an amber bottle with a spray top, so you can diffuse it evenly over your face when the day is wearing short and your spirits need gentle reviving.

Rose absolute is obtained when roses are extracted through the enfluerage method. This reddish liquid is just the remedy for emotional imbalances, reminding us to love ourselves. It also draws other love toward us. Try painting a small heart with a dab of rose absolute on the skin over your own heart and rubbing it in. Rose absolute adds a lovely note to a personal essence, especially with a small piece of rose quartz added to the bottom of the bottle.

I add rose otto to a night facial oil as an occasional luxurious ritual. I keep my small bottle of rose otto in a little wooden box my brother gave me. All I need to do is open the lid to inhale its sweet perfume. This oil, with the addition of marjoram, is also helpful in working through grief. Treat yourself and someone you love to a bottle of rose absolute or otto. Just a little dab can have a great effect on body, mind, and spirit.

Blending: Combining jasmine absolute with rose absolute creates the sweetest bath salts on earth. A few drops of sandalwood added to this blend can turn a bath into a sensual, sweet, calming experience.

ROSE GERANIUM *(Pelargonium graveolens)*

Nature: Rose geranium is another essential oil that people have strong feelings about: They either like it a lot, or they do not! Some change their feelings very suddenly. I have a friend who didn't like rose geranium at all, yet it seemed to be just the oil she needed. I let her take her time adjusting to its scent by suggesting only a small amount at a time. That was five years ago, and now she buys up to four ounces at a time of the best rose geranium I can find — she loves it! When she feels a bit off kilter, she adds six to eight drops of rose geranium to a warm bath. She is on hormone replacement therapy and rose geranium is believed to contain phyto, or plant hormones, that can help the human body's hormone system function properly. Research is

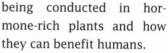

SUGGESTED RECIPE FOR ROSE GERANIUM

As bug repellent: Add 5 drops of rose geranium oil, 1 drop of peppermint oil, and 1 drop of lemongrass oil to 4 ounces of water. Place in a spray bottle and spray clothes before you go for a walk in the woods.

being conducted in hormone-rich plants and how they can benefit humans.

The scented geranium plant is lovely to look at, although its flowers are small. The essential oil is obtained from the leaf. There are many different kinds of scented geraniums, and I enjoy the various rose ones. The smell is an herbal/floral one. I find lemon geraniums delightful as well, but rose is the only one from which I have experienced the essential oil.

Benefits: Rose geranium is believed to be antidepressant, sedative, antiseptic, antidiabetic, uplifting and balancing, and insect repellant. The oil has been found useful in cases of depression, PMS, skin problems, neuralgia, and nervous tension.

Suggested Uses: Rose geranium is added to skin-care products, and can benefit all skin types. It is an excellent bath additive.

Rose geranium oil is a must for many women who need help balancing during those up and down hormonal times.

This oil has a reputation as an insect repellant, and is much more pleasant than some commercial products. Its effectiveness is enhanced when a small amount of peppermint or lemongrass is added. Always wash hands after applying essential oils, and keep hands away from the eyes.

Blending: Rose geranium can quickly overpower a blend. Keep this in mind when adding it to bath, body-care, and perfume oils. It blends well with other oils including lavender, bergamot, clary sage, patchouli, and lemon.

ROSEMARY (Rosmarinus officinalis)

Nature: Rosemary is a beautiful plant to grow and a most necessary essential oil for every home. It is traditionally associated with "remembrance," and was widely used at both weddings and funerals for centuries. Rosemary was burned as an incense in sick rooms to clear the air. I tucked a sprig in my father's casket when he passed away. My beloved kitty is named Rosemary — I could never forget her! Tied on a wedding or gift package, its tradition for remembrance is kept alive. A sprig of the herb, or a drop of the pure essential oil says, "I remember."

Rosemary is also valued for its preservative properties, and was often used in foods during times before refrigeration. I love a sprig or two of fresh rosemary roasted with lamb.

Benefits: Rosemary has been found to be analgesic, antiseptic, circulatory, regulating, antispasmodic, astringent, and a cerebral stimulant. It has been found effective in cases of headache, mental fatigue, cellulite, dandruff, hair loss, and poor memory.

Suggested Uses: Rosemary was one of the first essential oils I got to know. Having long hair, I was aware that the herb rosemary kept it shiny and healthy. I was delighted to discover rosemary pure essential oil as an easier and faster method of highlighting and conditioning my mane. Moreover, its piercing aroma is also known as a stimulant and is indeed a bit of a "wake up call."

I like to combine rosemary with clary sage, patchouli, and jasmine absolute to make a hair oil to add drop by drop to my wooden brush and comb (see recipe on page 137). The hair is protein in nature and readily absorbs pure essential oils. Their scent stays much longer in the hair than on the skin. This is my favorite place to wear a fragrance or perfume. The rosemary is what one first experiences and as it fades the jasmine, patchouli, and clary sage are left to linger.

Rosemary has been found to also ease stiff, aching, tired, or overworked muscles when used after activity as a massage or bath oil. It has been found to ease rheumatic and arthritic conditions when used in a massage oil. In cleaning water it revives the house *and* the maid! I love rosemary in a bath or shower soap to liven up my morning.

Rosemary essential oil can provide a much needed lift during a long day. Unlike coffee or other stimulants, it

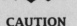

CAUTION

Rosemary can be irritating to the skin and must be properly diluted before any application to the skin.

Rosemary's sharp aroma has also been employed in inhalations for asthma and bronchitis. However, caution must be used as some prone to asthma are bothered by any scent that is too strong. Caution must also be observed when using rosemary with anyone prone to epilepsy.

doesn't boomerang and end up depleting energy. If I must keep evening appointments it provides a pick-me-up. It is most helpful in a simmer pot or diffuser when concentration and alertness are required.

I had some nursing students come to me for help in improving their memory skills prior to their board exams. We combined rosemary with two other cerebral stimulants, lemon and peppermint. They smelled the blend only when they studied and at no other time until the test day. When test day came, the nursing students took scented cotton balls with them, and sniffed their way to a very good score. They happily reported that they felt quite confident that the blend of pure essential oils did the trick to open up locked files in their brains when test nerves began to take over.

ROSEWOOD *(Aniba rosaeodora)*

Nature: Rosewood comes from a tree in the Brazilian rain forests, which is why some people decide to forgo its use. It has a very unique woodsy/floral scent which I love. I find it most useful for the skin and for its balancing effect, which is similar to that of rose geranium. It was once called "Bois de Rose," but isn't found under this name very often today.

Benefits: Rosewood is believed to be balancing, emotionally regenerating, antiseptic, soothing without being sedative, and cell regenerating. It has been found effective in cases of PMS, stress, skin care, headache, depression, nausea, anxiety, and tension.

Suggested Uses: Rosewood reminds me of the wonderful facials I experienced under the skillful hands of Magda Moursi, who has used essential oils in her skin-care salon for many years. If and when you can, indulge yourself in a professional facial. It does wonders for your skin and your soul. When you can't employ a facialist, at least employ pure essential oils in your personal home skin-care routine. Try rosewood in a blend with frankincense and lavender for an every-other-evening facial oil. All three oils are cell regenerating, and produce a wonderful smell just before bedtime.

Rosewood is also nice in hair care: Try blending it into a hair oil, or adding a few drops to a hairbrush before use for a refreshing experience.

I am quite fond of adding rosewood to blends for a special note to round them out. It is great in bath products.

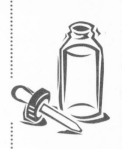

SANDALWOOD *(Santalum album)*

Nature: Sandalwood oil didn't impress me when I first experienced its nutty/woody fragrance. Now, years later, I would never be without my deep, sweet, sensuous, spiritually alive sandalwood. Its scent clings like a guardian angel to protect from life's evils. It is soothing to body, mind, and spirit.

Benefits: Sandalwood is believed to be antiseptic, moisturizing to the skin, antidepressant, expectorant, and aphrodisiac. It has been found effective in cases of dry skin, bronchitis, nervous tension, anxiety, and depression.

Suggested Uses: This ancient scent has perfumed many religious temples throughout time. I have a carved sandalwood bead necklace. I rub the oil into it neat and savor this luscious scent throughout the day. Sandalwood is a great scent for men!

SUGGESTED RECIPES FOR SANDALWOOD

For bronchitis: Add 6 drops to the water of a simmer pot for soothing relief.

For hair care: Add neat to hair ends to smooth them, provide a sweet sandalwood scent all day long.

For sore throat: Rub the oil neat into the neck area.

For Earth's Essence™ potpourri: In a large glass bowl (don't use wood or plastic, which absorb and retain scent), combine equal parts sandalwood chips, patchouli leaves, lavender buds, blue malva, oakmoss, juniper berries, and cinnamon chips or sticks. In a small bowl, combine 2 tablespoons each powdered sandalwood and cinnamon, or any combination of powdered spices to equal 2 tablespoons. Add 10 drops of sandalwood oil, 5 drops of patchouli oil, 1 drop of cinnamon oil, 5 drops of lavender oil, 3 drops of juniper oil, and 3 drops of vetiver oil. Make sure the oils are well-distributed by crushing all of the small lumps in the powder.

Add the oiled powder mixture to the herb mixture in the large bowl and mix well. Store in an airtight container (preferably glass) for a minimum of 2 weeks, shaking often to mix the herbs and powder well. Try filling a small cloth bag or an old sock with the mixture and hanging it in your car. When the scent begins to fade, toss the bag up on the dash, turn the heater vent on high for a few minutes, and savor the scent.

Blending: Sandalwood adds body to a blend, and adds to its staying power. It works particularly well in skin-care blends. In a massage oil, sandalwood clings to the skin like a protective film, leaving the recipient with a reminder to relax long after the massage is over. My Earth Essence™ potpourri is redolent of sandalwood, and has been known to last more than ten years (see recipe on previous page).

Caution: Sandalwood takes many years to grow and with the current demand for the oil it has the potential of becoming endangered and expensive. The oil is distilled from the heart wood of the sandalwood tree and it does not grow in very many places in the world. Mysore sandalwood, from a region in India by the same name, is rumored to have some of the finest qualities from which to distill essential oil. You can contact one of the associations listed on pages 338–339 to obtain more information on the possibly endangered status of this fine tree. Luckily, with sandalwood's lingering nature, a very small amount has a lasting effect.

TEA TREE *(Melaleuca alternifolia)*

Nature: This essential oil is distilled from a tree in Australia, and derives its name from its use as a tea by the aboriginal people. It is a medicinally scented oil that has a place in every household. Whenever my daughter walks into the house and smells the scent of tea tree she asks, "Who's sick, Mom?" It is one of those desert island oils like lavender that I would never be without.

Tea tree is safe to use neat on the most delicate parts of the body and has been successfully employed during war times when medicines were in short supply. This oil is gaining popularity as an ingredient in personal care products.

Benefits: Tea tree is fungicidal, antiseptic, expectorant, anti-infectious, anti-inflammatory, parasiticide, and antiviral.

Suggested Uses: This a head-to-toe oil that can be used to treat everything from dandruff to athlete's foot. I have experienced a few very nasty spider bites, complete with massive swelling and inflammation. When the medical community offered me little care for these, a combination of tea tree and lavender essential oils applied neat or undiluted to the area helped clear up the bites without scarring.

Yeast infections are very short-lived after antibiotic use of a tampon moistened with ten to fifteen drops of tea tree oil, used daily for seven days. There is *no* other essential oil that I would recommend applying in this manner. Other fungal infections like ringworm and athlete's foot respond well to the tea tree. It also helps heal scrapes, burns, and cuts. I have used it in a simmer pot of water to inhale during times of bronchial congestion.

VANILLA OLEORESIN *(Vanilla planifolia)*, or Absolute

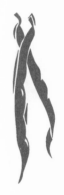

Nature: This easily recognizable orchid scent is a favorite of many folks. The true vanilla oleoresin or absolute is so deep, sweet, and wonderful that I include it in my Love Oil!

Vanilla blends great with most other oils, but it will settle to the bottom of a blend and therefore must be shaken well before use. This scent was often used as a perfume during the Depression. I still make vanilla perfume today and use it as a base for many other perfume blends.

Benefits: Vanilla is rarely disliked, in fact it has been shown to be one of the most popular scents known. It tends to remind us of homey feelings like baking cookies and warm feelings. Many find its scent relaxing.

Suggested Uses: Vanilla is a great bath additive, however it tends to sink to the bottom of the tub and has to be well dispersed. I often add it to bath salts instead of directly to the bath water. It also makes a nice addition to massage oils and personal essences in small amounts. These products must be shaken well and often. Vanilla's main aromatherapeutic value is that everyone usually likes it, more than any actual chemical properties it has to help enable us to feel better. Vanilla is one of those scents that once you experience the true scent, the imitations pale in comparison.

YLANG-YLANG *(Cananga odorata)*

Nature: People love to pronounce the name of this pure essential oil. I've heard lang-lang, e-lang-e-lang, and a few other variations. What is important is that the name means "flower of flowers."

Benefits: Ylang-ylang is believed to be antidepressant, aphrodisiac, sedative, calming, euphoric, antiseptic, and hypotensive. It has been found effective in reducing sexual difficulties resulting from anxiety, stress, and depression. The oil has also been used for cases of rapid heart beat, depression, frigidity, impotence, high blood pressure, and nervous tension.

Suggested Uses: Ylang-ylang is so sweet that it can be overpowering; it must be used in small amounts and high dilutions. I like to use it in baths, relaxing massage oils, skin-care oils, and bath salts. My daughter, who generally finds essential oils too strong for her taste, likes ylang-ylang. When she was younger, I used to put just a drop in her evening bath and she enjoyed it.

My sister found ylang-ylang helpful during her pregnancy when high blood pressure threatened. The scent calmed and relaxed her, which naturally lowered her blood pressure. She added two drops to her humidifier. (Use caution when adding pure essential oils to any thing with plastic internal parts, since too much oil can damage the plastic. However, a few drops twice a day shouldn't hurt.)

I once knew a man who loved this oil so much that he wore it like cologne. I never thought of it as a masculine oil, but he certainly changed my view on that — it works equally well for men and women. How about a candlelight bath for two! With the addition of some soft music and an open mind, wonderful things could result. Try an inhalation, a diffuser, or massage to employ this oil exotically.

Brushing ylang-ylang oil through the hair is a wonderful experience. Remember, only a drop or two is ever needed. Higher concentrations could result in headache or nausea.

Blending: Ylang-ylang can be just the right oil to add a sweet, relaxing note to a blend. I, again, caution about its odor intensity. With ylang-ylang, as with other pure essential oils, one must remember that you can always add more but it is impossible to take them out, so less is best.

Ylang-ylang and lavender baths are one of life's little pleasures. The addition of sandalwood or rose enhances the experience even more.

LESS COMMONLY USED PURE ESSENTIAL OILS

These oils are less commonly used because the general public doesn't have much information about their potential uses. Some of these oils — linden, labdanum, and yarrow — are rare, others are potentially dangerous if improperly used, like hyssop and cinnamon. I include this selected group because I have found beneficial uses for them in my life.

BENZOIN *(Styrax benzoin)*

Nature: This resin has been recognized as a purifier by ancient cultures and is believed to drive away bad energy and evil spirits. Many cultures believed that sweet scents sent heavenward would incur the blessings of their gods. Benzoin has a warm vanilla-like scent. It has been used for centuries in incense and as a preservative in cosmetics. This resinous compound sunk and actually adhered solidly to my bathtub when I used it in a bath to help combat depression.

Benefits: Benzoin has been found to help retain skin elasticity. It is valuable in treating dry cracked skin, and is believed to be antidepressant, anti-inflammatory, antiseptic, an expectorant and sedative.

Suggested Uses: I add benzoin to my nail-care formulas. It works wonderfully to clear up dry ragged cuticles and condition the surrounding skin. Benzoin is excellent as a fixative in a personal essence and very relaxing and soothing in a bath blend or incense.

CEDARWOOD, ATLAS *(Cedrus atlantica)*

Nature: This is not the cedarwood that reminds us of standing at the pencil sharpener in school or that lines the gerbil cage. The scent is different, not so strong or so pencil-like! The cedarwoods of Texas and Virginia do produce a different pure essential oil that is used as insect repellent, is a powerful abortifacient (can cause abortion), and has some aromatherapeutic properties. However, for home use Atlas cedarwood is preferred. It can be soothing, and is used in cosmetics, incense, and household products.

Benefits: Atlas cedarwood is believed to be sedative, an expectorant, antiseptic, astringent, and antiseborrhoeic (balancing to the production of sebum — a secretion from the sweat glands).

Suggested Uses: Add a few drops to a hair care blend. This isn't as overwhelming in scent as other cedar woods, and blends well with sandalwood, juniper, patchouli, jasmine absolute, rosemary, and clary sage — all essential oils that complement a hair blend. I blend it in hair blends for clients with dandruff problems, or hair loss.

Sometimes, I will put Atlas cedarwood in a simmer pot to soothe a bronchial problem. It is also fungicidal and is nice in a spray to help control mold and mildew. I add it to my mop water. Try applying some to your tent before you put it away for the season by adding a few drops to water, spray on, and let dry. Patchouli or tea tree blend would work well for this, too.

CINNAMON BARK *(Cinnamomum zeylanicum)*

Nature: Extreme caution must be observed with spicy, hot cinnamon. Be very careful to avoid contact with mucous membranes and eyes. I never use this oil on my body, although others do in a very high dilution. Although true cinnamon essential oil can be caustic to the skin and expensive, it is preferable to the synthetic cinnamon scents available.

Benefits: Cinnamon is best used to scent the environment. A blend of two drops of cinnamon, ten drops of patchouli, and ten drops of lavender mixed with eight ounces of water in a spray bottle makes a superb home air freshener. This formula is antifungal and really makes a musty old basement a nicer place to work. I spray this on my basement stairs and in dark corners that don't get much air circulation or light. The scent lingers and has a spicy, earthy, clean scent. Be careful not to spray on yourself or pets.

A great winter holiday scent is two drops of cinnamon oil blended with ten drops of pine, fir, or juniper oil in water to scent the home for the holidays. Try spraying this blend on carpeting or adding it to a simmer pot. Cinnamon and sweet orange also makes a nice spicy home fragrance.

CYPRESS (Cupressus sempervirens)

Nature: There are several different species of cypress being distilled for an essential oil. This species yields a superior-quality essential oil. Cypress has a pleasant scent that blends well with other essential oils like juniper, bergamot, pine, cedarwood, or lavender. It is a seldom-used essential oil, but very effective when employed. The Tibetan people find cypress purifying and burn it as an incense.

Benefits: Cypress is believed to be astringent, deodorant, styptic, antiseptic, antispasmodic, and vasoconstrictive.

Suggested Uses: Cypress is great in a foot bath or powder for sweaty feet. It has been used to make a soothing oil for varicose veins (to be applied, not massaged in). Cypress also helps stem the flow of excessive perspiration in a deodorant blend, and eases heavy mentrual periods when applied as a compress to the abdominal area. I add two drops to a simmer pot to breathe in when I have a cough. Adding a few drops in a pet's bath deodorizes and repels fleas.

FRANKINCENSE *(Boswellia carteri)*

Nature: Frankincense has a unique, sweet balsamlike scent. It is a favorite for inhalations and has enjoyed a centuries-old reputation as an incense to cleanse and purify a home or temple. The scent of this fine essential oil is a bonus to its cell-regenerating properties. I love to just smell this precious liquid right from the bottle, and often burn the resin form along with myrrh in my home. Frankincense can be expensive, but the pure essential oil is very much worth the cost and is one I always have on hand.

Benefits: Frankincense is believed to be antiseptic, cytophylactic, anti-inflammatory, and sedative, and an expectorant.

Suggested Uses: I have found frankincense or the "true" incense essential oil to be very valuable as an inhalation for treating bronchitis. The sweet stream swirling up from the simmer pot eases breathing and the spirit.

In a mature-skin blend, frankincense can't be beat. I love to blend it with rose otto, lavender, and sandalwood in a calendula oil base for a facial oil. I also employ frankincense in a body lotion for arms and legs that have been overexposed to the sun. It's pampering, protecting, and comforting.

As a bath oil, frankincense blends well with floral and citrus oils, and deep, long-lasting scented oils like patchouli, sandalwood, or vetiver, a deeply grounding and calming oil distilled from a scented grass. I also add it to a bath with juniper when I feel overburdened. Frankincense is a nice addition to a personal essence blend.

HYSSOP *(Hyssopus officinalis)*
Nature: Opening, tonic, stimulating effect to the respiratory system, antiseptic.
Benefits: This oil isn't in common use, although it is invaluable in pulmonary conditions. I found hyssop most valuable last winter when I had a bout with bronchitis. I added three drops to a simmer pot with six drops each of sandalwood and lavender to help clear my lungs, which were quite tight and congested. After taking a few breaths over the warm simmer pot, I felt relief in my chest. I also added this blend to two ounces of sweet almond oil and used it to massage my chest between inhalations, three times per day. Accompanied by inhalations from a sniffy bag, this treatment helped get me on the road back to health quickly.
Caution: Hyssop should never be used with people prone to epileptic seizures because it has been found powerful enough to trigger a seizure. Hyssop can also be difficult to find, so you may have to find a mail-order source.

LABDANUM *(Cistus ladaniferus)*
Nature: This oil yields from a variety of the rock rose. It was once collected in the wild by scraping it off the beards of wandering goats grazing in the Grecian Islands. It is not in common use, yet is so unique that I am compelled to include it.
Suggested Uses: I suggest using labdanum oil in an alcohol-based perfume blend as it dissolves and blends better. It adds a deep note to a personal essence and also acts as a fixative to hold the scent. This resinous oil will stain clothing so use caution if adding it to a blend to wear as a personal essence. Labdanum was employed by the ancients as a fumigant to clear the air. The scent is similar to ambergris, a waxy substance secreted from whales, found floating in oceans, and used as a perfume fixative.

Ambergris (sometimes referred to as amber oil) and other animal-derived substances such as civet and musk were once popular as perfume ingredients though they are rarely, if ever, found in use or commerce today.

LINDEN BLOSSOM (Tilia vulgaris)

Nature: With its sweet, wonderful honeylike fragrance, I love linden in personal essence blends. It is sometimes referred to as lime blossom or lime tree.

Benefits: Linden is a nervine, sedative, and tonic. It seems to elicit a calming influence upon the user and aids in reducing nervous tension. Linden blossom has also been found effective as a soothing and softening agent when added to skin-care products.

MANDARIN (Citrus nobilis or madurensis)

Nature: Mandarin is a citrus-scented, sweet, tangy delight. The Italian fruit is suppose to yield a superior essential oil. Mandarin may be photo-toxic and sun exposure must be avoided after use. The scent is refreshing, uplifting, and revitalizing.

Benefits: One of mandarin's greatest benefits is its gentleness. Children love this essential oil and it is gentle enough to be included in their lives. Mandarin is also believed safe to use during pregnancy, so it could be employed by an expectant mother to enhance her household a bit. It is believed to discourage stretch marks when blended with lavender, sandalwood, and frankincense in a good base oil or combination including wheat germ oil. This oil is gentle for the aged too. Even PMS sufferers have found mandarin may ease their distress. It blends well with lavender.

Suggested Uses: A mandarin-scented bath is great when one is feeling blue. Follow it up with a massage with mandarin in the massage oil. Mandarin is a nice part of an uplifting personal essence. Children's rooms and school bags can be freshened with a wipe-down of mandarin in water. An evening massage can be a special treat for a child after homework is done.

Try combining one to two drops of mandarin in two ounces of witch hazel for a refreshing facial or body toner to apply with cotton buds.

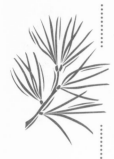

PINE *(Pinus sylvestris)*, also called Scots or Norwegian Pine

Nature: There are many pines that yield an essential oil, but not all are useful on aromatherapy. This pine is safer than some cruder distillates. The scent of real pine is so superior to any synthetic creation that I cannot understand why more folks don't use real pine instead of the dreadful imitations. Pine has been recognized as a healing tree ever since humans first discovered that a walk in a pine forest invigorated and decongested. Pine is synonymous with "clean." Its needles and essential oil have been used to disinfect castle and cottage alike.

Benefits: Pine is believed to help clear the mind and clean the environment. It has been employed as an antiviral, antiseptic, expectorant, restorative, and stimulant.

Suggested Uses: I very seldom use pine in a bath or massage oil because it can cause skin irritation. When I do, I use very little and save it for those times when I need a deep refreshing. It also is an essential oil I tend to use more in winter. There is no better scent for the holidays than pine and cinnamon bark, unless it's Siberian fir and cinnamon bark. Add them to a simmer pot or put a few drops of the blend on cotton and tuck them around the house. Both pine and cinnamon can be dermal irritants, so use an eyedropper and wash your hands after handling them. Remember they can mar plastic surfaces. You can also make carpet freshener with these oils to scent the house for a holiday party.

I like pine best when I have the chore of cleaning the house and I am weary. Ten to fifteen drops of pine oil in soapy water can make the task a lot easier and much more beneficial to the housekeeper. The imitation pine cleaners pale in comparison.

ROMAN CHAMOMILE *(Chamaemelum nobile)*

Nature: Roman chamomile is distilled from a certain type of chamomile flower, either Roman or German *(Matricaria recutica)*. Roman is clear and sweet whereas German is usually a deep blue/green color and has a much more bitter scent.

Benefits: Chamomile is believed to be analgesic, anti-inflammatory, antispasmodic, and a nerve sedative.

Suggestions for Use: Chamomile oil is a must for headache sufferers. Blend two drops of Roman chamomile oil with five drops of lavender oil in a large bowl of warm water. Take a small cloth towel and barely skim the surface of this mixture with it; apply the warm compress to your aching head. I've found that this treatment in a dark, quiet room works when all else fails. Chamomile oil also works well on sunburn when blended with lavender oil. Taken in tea form, the herb chamomile has a long-standing folk reputation for promoting relaxation and a good night's sleep. It is mild and pleasant to the taste. Be sure to steep the tea for no more than three minutes or it becomes bitter. If this occurs, strain the tea and use it to cleanse your skin or rinse through your hair for added shine. When traveling, I carry a small 2 ml bottle of Roman chamomile in my backpack and inhale deeply of its essence whenever I feel weary. Chamomile herb and oils also make soothing baths. Two drops each of Roman chamomile and lavender oils make a relaxing evening bath. Six drops of this precious essence diffused in a simmer pot of water during times of great stress can transform the mood in the room from harried and stressed to much more tranquil and manageable. This is a good addition to the headache compress treatment for an especially stubborn headache.

Roman chamomile is gentle and effective for children's baths and massage oils when used well diluted. One drop of oil to ½ ounce base is sufficient. The scent is sweet and comforting.

THYME *(Thymus vulgaris)*
Benefits: Thyme is believed to be antiseptic, an expectorant, nervine, antispasmodic, and carminative.
Suggestions for Use: Thyme is a very potent oil and no more than a drop or two is ever needed. Add it to a simmer pot with frankincense and hyssop to clear the air and ease breathing. This pure essential oil was very valuable to me during a bout with bronchitis.

YARROW *(Achillea millefolium)*
Nature: This often hard-to-obtain oil is worth the effort and funds spent in acquiring it. I have distilled this precious herb and found it delightful to watch its azure blue pure essential oil form on the filter paper.
Benefits: Yarrow has similar properties to chamomile. It is believed to be anti-inflammatory, antispasmodic, hypotensive, and carminative.

Suggestions for Use: Use yarrow water like a rosewater for skin. This is the water left from distilling the white yarrow flowers. It is quite wild and strong-smelling, much more like the smell of the flower than that of the pure essential oil. The distillation process is time-consuming and produces small yields. (I garnered approximately ten drops after working for three days and nights gathering armloads of wild yarrow in nearby fields and distilling the flower tops.) You could make a yarrow water similar to the recipe I give for rosewater, by adding two drops yarrow oil to a four-ounce bottle of spring or distilled water. Remember to keep this refrigerated and use it as quickly as possible because it has no preservatives. This preparation will smell much sweeter than the by-product yarrow water obtained from the distilling process.

Yarrow has been respected as a healing herb since ancient times. I have used yarrow's anti-inflammatory properties to soothe sunburn by adding five drops of beautiful blue yarrow pure essential oil and five drops of lavender oil to a four-ounce spray bottle of spring water. This mixture can also be added to a cream base to soothe onto the skin. The scent of yarrow oil is very unique and the natural blue hue it adds to skin care products is beautiful.

CAUTION:
ESSENTIAL OILS TO AVOID

There are a number of essential oils that are best to avoid using altogether. These oils can be toxic and have little value for the home enthusiast.

Almond	Lavender Cotton	Pennyroyal	Southernwood
Bitter Birch	Mugwort	Rue	Tansy
Boldo Leaf	Mustard	Sage	Thuja
Calamus	Onion	Sassafras	Wintergreen
Cassia	Oregano	Savine	Wormseed
Horseradish	Orrisroot	Savory	Wormwood

LEARNING HOW TO USE ESSENTIAL OILS

You may be eager and ready to learn about essential oils, but don't know where to begin. It is very possible — and enjoyable — to explore and learn about the world of essential oils on your own, or informally with a group of friends.

Following are some questions you can use to learn more about individual pure essential oils on your own. Inhale the particular pure essential oil you're exploring and answer the following questions about it.

◆ How do you feel when you smell this aroma?
◆ What do you think it would be beneficial in healing?
◆ Where on your body would you like to put this oil, if anywhere?
◆ Which part of the plant do you think this oil comes from?
◆ How does this oil affect you? Close your eyes, inhale deeply, then record how this experience made you feel emotionally, or what you saw as a result.
◆ Does this essential oil remind you of anything or any place? Make a list of these associations.
◆ What would you like to blend this oil with?
◆ Which part of the earth do you think this oil comes from?
◆ Is the oil masculine or feminine to you, or both?
◆ Is this essence hot or cold?
◆ List several words that best describe this aroma.

Go to your books and study guides to learn as much as possible about this particular oil. Then answer the following questions to the best of your ability. Throughout your exploration, remember to enjoy this process of learning about nature's bounty.

◆ What is the essential oil's name?
◆ What is its botanical name?
◆ What is its country of origin?
◆ Name a few chemical constituents of this essential oil.
◆ What is the odor intensity of this oil?
◆ What is the suggested dilution? In which base oils?
◆ Are there similar oils? Which ones?
◆ What does this oil blend best with?
◆ What are the traditional uses for this oil?
◆ What is the safety data on this oil?
◆ How can you incorporate it into your lifestyle?

CHAPTER 12
Basic Blending Advice

Before you can begin blending and using essential oils, you need to set up a work area. I have a back room of my home set aside for my work area, although my essential oils are stored in the cool, dark basement. I must go up and down the stairs often, but consider this good exercise. You must figure out which area of your home or business will best suit your needs and taste. I prefer the back room because it is away from the hustle and bustle of the main house and is a bit cooler and quieter place, where I can concentrate and work. Good ventilation is important, especially when working for prolonged amounts of time with essential oils. They can become quite overpowering when used in a closed area. I like to run a small fan when working for longer than an hour in an enclosed area. A cool work area is also beneficial. I try to never bottle in direct sunlight, or in a very hot room where the essential oils can quickly evaporate. A flat, even surface that is uncluttered is best. I have had accidental spills that ruined paperwork, labels, and other products.

Easy access to hot water is a must. You'll need to be able to clean your hands and glass equipment such as beakers and bottles with hot soapy water. Some clients have had success cleaning their bottles in a very hot dishwasher — with the pleasant side effect of a lovely smelling home. You will need accessible shelving for storing oils and bases. Arranging the bottles in alphabetical order makes it easier to find what you're looking for quickly and know when it's time to reorder a particular oil.

EQUIPMENT AND SUPPLIES

The equipment and supplies you need to begin experimenting with essential oils are simple to acquire and assemble.

The most expensive supplies will, of course, be the pure essential oils you choose to experiment with. The bases can also be expensive, depending on which ones you prefer. I suggest trying just a few oils and bases in small quantities to start, and get to know them well. To begin, 4 to 10 ml of pure essential oils and 1 to 4 ounces of base oils are sufficient to experiment with in blending small batches.

The piece of equipment that can be expensive is an aromatic diffuser, averaging from $29 to $100, depending upon the model. Oshadhi/R.J.F. Inc. and Aroma Vera in California offer wonderful lines of diffusers (see Resources).

For Blending and Storing Oils

Clean dark glass bottles. Collect a variety of sizes from 1 dram (4 ml) to 8 ounces (236 ml). Well-washed old vitamin and tincture bottles work well. This is a good chance to fill those pretty perfume bottles everyone seems to have, but doesn't know what to put in them. Make a perfume to go with the bottle and give it as a gift.

Plastic should be used only as temporary storage for any herb or spice. It is porous enough to allow precious essential oils to penetrate and dissipate into the air. Dark, tightly stoppered or capped, glass bottles are always the ideal storage for herbs and spices and essential oils.

Glass beakers and glass mixing rods. Glass beakers with milliliter measurements are helpful for measuring oils and blends to proper proportions. The lips on the beakers make pouring much easier. I was given my set by a faithful work-study student who worked as a chemist. These are available through biological and chemist supply businesses, which are often found in college towns. Medical supply houses also carry beakers, as well as droppers for measuring pure essential oils. Pharmacies often have bottles and droppers available or a pharmacist may be able to refer you to a source. Bottle companies often have large minimum orders and aren't useful for the home blender. Frontier Cooperative Herbs (see Resources) offers bottles and droppers in any quantity and a variety of sizes. They also sell a 4-ounce amber spray bottle that is perfect for making personal spray blends or perfumes. Aromaland (see Resources) also offers good-quality dark amber glass bottles, dropper top bottles, eyedroppers, and aroma lamps. I have had success finding out-of-state suppliers in phone books available in my local library.

Base oils. You will need sweet almond, jojoba, and grapeseed oils for diluting pure essential oils before use.

As I said earlier, 1 to 4 ounces is a good quantity to have on hand to start. I use an average of 8 ounces of sweet almond oil in a month for after-shower rubs, hair oil treatments, bath oils, and my personal massage oils. The amounts I use of other base oils such as jojoba, evening primrose, calendula, apricot kernel, or grapeseed depends on the products I'm producing.

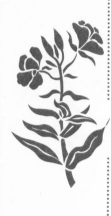

Base oils are available in quantities from 1 ounce to usually 16 ounces in health food stores, co-ops, and even in some grocery stores. I personally prefer to order them from a reputable supplier rather than chance buying a bottle off a store shelf that has gone rancid. Often I will ask the proprietor how long the oil has been on the shelf, and don't hesitate to return a rancid oil. Rancid base oils are commonly found on store shelves, and are identifiable by their off smell. Most base oils have only a light scent or barely any scent at all. When a base oil is rancid, the off-smell can overpower the scent of the essential oil added to it, and should not be used. I try to use all base oils within three to six months of purchase.

I add 1 tablespoon of wheat germ oil to every 2 ounces of massage or body oil I make that requires an extended shelf life (more than three months). I also add 10 drops of pure vitamin E (approximately three punctured capsules) for every 2 ounces of base. I very seldom make up blends in advance unless they are to be put on a store shelf or sold at a craft show. I inform my customers that these are to be used as soon as possible and to smell them closely before using if they have been left longer than six months.

Wash items such as massage table sheets, towels, and robes or clothes that come in contact with base oils as soon as possible in very hot soapy water. Buy only what you can use in the near future to avoid using rancid oils.

Sea salt. This is a great base for bath salts. It's also a very economical way to experience one of the precious, costly essential oils since you only need to add a drop or two of oil to a couple cups (approximately 500 ml) of sea salt. I like to mix both coarse and fine grinds. I purchase 5-pound bags of both coarse and fine grinds and blend them in equal parts myself. To make salt glow, only fine grind should be used.

Sea salt is soothing to soak in and looks lovely with small amounts of herbs or flowers added along with the pure essential oils and absolutes. Just make sure the salt is well dissolved in the bath water or you will end up sitting on uncomfortable sharp little lumps. Remember to keep those precious crystals well stoppered to prevent the volatile essential oils and absolutes from escaping into the environment and reducing the potency and effects of the bath salts. Also, salt naturally absorbs moisture so keeping the salts well-sealed prevents this and helps keep the mixture from becoming lumpy.

Labels. You need to label every bottle with the ingredients, date of creation, and directions for use. Here's a chance to use your creativity — handmade labels greatly enhance an essential oil collection. For many years, I hand rubber-stamped all of the labels on my products. I created scenes with the sun, butterflies, bees, trees, clouds, stars, moons, flowers, and little animals — and palm trees and dolphins for the citrus oil blends!

The computer opens up all kinds of new possibilities. With the right software, the possibilities are endless.

Stickers add a nice accent to a bottle of essential oil. Victorian motifs with flowers, ferns, lovely ladies, and gardens look great against a dark amber glass bottle. It's fun to search for special stickers that fit the person or occasion for which the oil is being made.

A special handwritten label makes the bottle of blended oils more personal. I like to use gold, silver, or white paint pens to label a special bottle. Just be sure to use ink that won't smear if it comes into contact with the oils. Petroleum-based inks tend to run.

Glass eyedroppers. The rubber tops of these will eventually break down from contact with the pure essential oils. To avoid this, try to collect pure essential oils with dropper top bottles; otherwise, do your best to keep the oil off of the rubber bulb of the glass eyedropper.

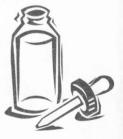

For Diffusing Oils

Spray bottles. Collect a variety of sizes from 4 ounces to 16 ounces. These come in handy for everything from spritzing rosewater upon your face to clearing the air in a pet's area. Spray bottles, when well shaken, will propel pure essential oils and water over the body, home, or vehicle. If reusing one of these, make sure it is positively clean and does not contain residue of a toxic substance. I often buy new ones for healing blends I'm planning to spray on the body, and reuse old ones for home cleaning or car care blends.

Diffuser. Aromatic diffusers contain a little glass nebulizer attached to an air pump, much like an aquarium motor. Working without heat, the pump on this electronic device blends air and pure essential oils and sprays a fine mist out into the room. I have seen and tried many prototypes of these little machines, yet rarely use one. One innovative colleague sent me a battery-operated diffuser with an attachment for my belt. I can't imagine needing oils around me that much! The rare times I do use a diffuser are when I need to get a large amount of oils into the air but do not want to heat them, such as when I'm sleeping or not available to keep an eye on the candle and simmer pot.

I know people who swear by diffusers and wouldn't be without one. They can be expensive to buy and operate, depending on the pure essential oils one chooses to use. Many of the diffusers I tried actually were damaged by undiluted oils. The oils marred the plastic surfaces and the tubing had to be replaced. Some of the newer models have corrected this problem.

Use caution in choosing a place to set a diffuser. You don't want essential oil mist landing on valuable furniture surfaces it might mar. One advantage of diffusers is that they can be put on a timer. I once played around with making an aromatic alarm clock of rosemary and lemon timed to come on shortly before I had to rise. It was fun, although I am naturally quite time-sensitive and rarely need or use an alarm clock. Not everyone is so lucky. A "diffuser alarm" might be useful if you're a slow riser.

Simmer pot. Lately, these have become very popular gifts accompanied by a bag of simmering potpourri. They are available in most housewares departments of retail stores, and most craft shops. Prices range from $1 for a candle-heated model in the dollar store, up to $15 for an electric model, depending on the size. The simmer pot works by heating water containing essential oils, which are then diffused into the air. I fill the pot with water, then add the desired essential oils, but you must keep an eye on the water level. I have never had one get to the boiling point, but you must use caution to be sure the pot doesn't burn dry! The electric models can be put on a timer.

Simmer pots work well outdoors to drive away bugs, or in the house when someone is ill. Because the oils added to a simmer pot or an aromatic diffuser are undiluted, the effects are a bit stronger than oils first added to a base and then applied directly to the skin.

Aroma lamp. These are like simmer pots — minus the water. The pure essential oils are added directly to a warming area and diffused. These can be very elaborate in their designs. These are heated either with a candle or electrically and must be used with caution.

Lightbulb rings. I personally don't use lightbulb rings very often and have seen them catch fire if too much oil was placed on a hot light bulb. They are meant to be placed on a cold bulb, and filled before the light is turned on. I have had difficulty keeping them on the lamp or fitting them between the lamp and the shade. I also had problems with them arriving broken and/or cracked from suppliers so check yours carefully before purchase.

If you choose to use a lightbulb ring, I recommend a ceramic glazed one, rather than the floppy asbestos types. Unglazed ones simply absorb the essential oil, making it difficult to change scents. Rings with a small indentation for holding the oils work better.

Homemade diffusing equipment. If you don't want to invest in any special equipment to start with, you can diffuse essential oils right from your stove. I often add a few drops of pure essential oil to the pan of water I keep on my woodstove all winter. I have also scented a room using an old saucepan on top of the kitchen stove. Another place I add small amounts of essential oils (10 drops) is the humidifier on my furnace. When sickness threatens members of my household, I add eucalyptus, which works wonderfully to clear the air. Be cautious about using too much essential oil because it could cause damage to internal plastic parts. I reserve this practice for times when it's most necessary, not more than two to three times a winter.

Aroma jewelry. This has become quite popular recently, although I have collected aroma jewelry for more than 10 years. My collection includes several necklaces with compartments where pure essential oils can be added, and a pair of earrings with a place to add a few drops of oil. My favorite piece is a cherished gift called a posy pin. This is a small glass vase on a stick pin that can be filled with water so that small flowers and herbs can then be placed in it. I love to fill it with Johnny-jump up, lily-of-the-valley, miniature roses, spearmint, violets, thyme, lavender, chamomile flowers, and soapwort. This little treasure keeps the flowers fresh all day long and, when placed on my lapel, enables me to enjoy their scent wherever I go. Sometimes I also pin it on a hat.

BASE OILS

Carrier or base oils are the substances that pure essential oils are diluted into for making various preparations, including bath, body, facial, and massage products.

You may choose from a variety of bases, depending on individual needs and preferences. Bases like sweet almond, grapeseed, apricot kernel, avocado, or jojoba (which is actually liquid wax) are oily to the touch. You may also choose to use a cream or gel base. I use them all, depending on the type of skin care or treatment I'm making. Base oils like evening primrose, avocado, hazelnut, rosehip, and calendula can be expensive and are usually purchased and used in small amounts for special blends. I only buy 2 ounces at a time of these. The more common — and less expensive — base oils include sweet almond, grapeseed, and apricot kernel. I often purchase these by as much as a gallon.

Select a base that is as high a quality as your pure essential oils. There is no sense in putting fine oils into a synthetic or mineral oil base. Most essential oil companies carry a variety of bases, or you may choose to experiment with making your own. Many herbal skin-care books have recipes for making your own lotions and creams from natural, pure ingredients. Aloe vera gel can also be used when a cream or oil base isn't appropriate.

Following are some of the base ingredients you may want to have on hand for experimentation.

Apricot kernel oil. Full of vitamins and minerals, this oily base is good for skin-care products for all types of skin. It is especially useful on sensitive and aging skin. I refer to this as mature skin — which includes any skin that is more than 20 years old.

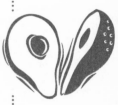

Avocado oil. This is nice as 10 percent of a facial oil. It is beneficial to all skins and contains vitamins and fatty acids.

Grapeseed oil. This oily base is much lighter to the touch than most others. It makes a nice massage oil alone, or combined with sweet almond oil. I like to use it for massaging the back because my hands seem to glide over a larger area easier. It is less viscous than other bases. The best grapeseed oil I ever obtained was fresh from a winery. Its green hue can be detected even in amber bottles.

Jojoba oil. This liquid wax solidifies when allowed to cool. It is an excellent base for personal essences because it doesn't "go off," or become rancid as quickly as some of the others. I use jojoba to extend costly essential oils such as rose, jasmine, sandalwood, and linden. A 10 percent dilution works well. I always list this dilution on my products so clients know the essential oil has been cut. Diluting in jojoba oil is a good avenue for allowing people to experience an oil at a lower cost than buying it undiluted.

Jojoba is nourishing to the skin and hair. I use ⅓ part jojoba oil in hair oils.

Sweet almond oil. Great base for massage, bath, body, and skin-care products. Sweet almond oil is scentless and nourishing to the skin. It relieves dry skin and may be used by itself, unscented, just to condition the skin. I like to apply it after a shower to my still-damp skin. It emulsifies with the water and blends in nicely. The addition of pure essential oils can make the almond oil a key part of an individual skin-care regime. I also combine it with jojoba oil for a hair oil treatment.

Wheat germ oil. Added in a 10 percent ratio to a skin-care product, this yellow oil helps extend the product's shelf life and benefits the skin with its high vitamin, mineral, and protein content.

Other bases. Essential oils may also be added to readymade products such as shampoo, conditioner, skin lotion, powder, dish soap, cleaning bases, as well as to water (for household sprays), alcohol (for perfumes), and sea salt.

MAKING YOUR OWN BLENDS

When working with a readymade product such as those listed above, start by adding very small amounts of essential oil to the base — only a drop or two per application — until you find a combination you like. Keep a pencil and pad of paper handy to record your experiments, successes, and failures. The best way to learn is to just start blending a little bit at a time. Abide by all cautions on working with essential oils (see pages 127–131) and let your nose, knowledge, and intuition be your guide. Picking up a few really good books on herbs and natural beauty will help too.

You will find guidelines on mixing and blending your own personal herbal and aromatic products at home in natural beauty books, herbals, and aromatherapy books. Look for books with an easy-to-understand format and that require ingredients that can be easily obtained. To identify useful books, ask friends if they have a tried and true favorite book. Reviews in holistic or herbal publications like the magazine, *The Herb Companion* (see Resources) may also be very helpful.

Another good way to experiment is with a group of friends. Have a day when you get together with friends and make an herbal facial steam, mask, and aromatherapy hair oil. Once you've made your products, trade massages and do a natural manicure and pedicure. These are life's little pleasures and a lot of fun to share, as well as beneficial to your health and beauty.

When blending, it's best to make up small batches that are fresh each time. Most of the bases you're blending the oils with aren't meant to have a long shelf life and contain none, or only

BODY OIL GIFT PACKAGING

Small bottles of fresh body and bath oils make great gifts. Begin with small (2 ounce) clear glass bottles. (A wide-mouth bottle makes it much easier to remove any spent plant material after the oil is used.) Fill each bottle with a base oil blend (including grapeseed and sweet almond), then add pure essential oils and a few nice dried flowers and herbs from the garden. Like all natural products, these bottles aren't meant to have a long shelf life; they should be used within four weeks.

Try mixing a variety of blends — I like to create a relaxing blend, an uplifting blend, a mature skin blend, a blend of patchouli, lavender, and rose absolute, and a plain lavender one. The oils I like using for these blends include lavender, rosewood, frankincense, rose absolute, patchouli, sweet orange, and clary sage. Vitamin E and wheatgerm oils are nice additions to some blends. For herbs and buds, I suggest rosebuds, lavender sprigs, calendula petals, rose hips, and California bay leaves.

Finish off the bottle with a nice label noting that the oil can be used as a floating bath oil, an after shower or bath moisturizing oil, or as a massage oil, and tie it with a ribbon around the neck of the bottle. It's a good idea also to include a note of caution about avoiding direct sunlight if the blend includes citrus oils like bergamot, sweet orange, and lemon. These are best for evening or indoor use.

a small amount of, natural preservative. Be sure to label what you have added and the date. Before using, always make sure that your products are well mixed and shaken so the pure essential oils are evenly distributed.

SOLUTIONS AND DILUTIONS

Solutions refer to the bases that one uses to blend the pure essential oils in, and the final product outcome. Dilutions refer to how much pure essential oil is incorporated into the solution. The solutions and dilutions you choose depend on individual needs and desired strength of the finished product. For instance, I would use a very small amount of pure essential oil in a cream or oil for the face, whereas a larger amount can be used in a cream for the less delicate skin of the arms or legs. A spray intended as a facial toner would have a much smaller concentration of pure essential oils than one intended to be used as a lingering perfume. This is why proper labeling is so very important!

One of the keys to using essential oils successfully is discovering what solution each oil is best dissolved in, and what dilution works best for your needs. This part of working with essential oils can get very exacting and mathematical, which is why this is the part that I am least enchanted with when it comes to using pure essential oils. If you have a propensity for math and calculating, you may enjoy this part. However, mathematical skills are not critical to success, and

---

USEFUL EQUIVALENCY MEASUREMENTS TO KNOW

◆ ½ fluid ounce = approximately 15 ml

◆ 1 percent solution = 5 drops essential oil in 4 teaspoons (20 ml) carrier oil

◆ 1 gram (a weight measurement) is approximately equal to 1 ml (a volume measurement)

◆ 1 gram or 1 ml equals approximately 20 drops of essence

SUGGESTED DILUTION FORMULAS

◆ 2 to 5 drops pure essential oil to 1 teaspoon carrier (1 teaspoon = 5 ml)

◆ 6 to 15 drops pure essential oil to 1 tablespoon carrier (1 tablespoon = 15 ml)

once you're quite familiar with the process, you can skip the math and begin to use your trained nose and intuition. But it's best to measure carefully and proceed cautiously when beginning.

I recommend beginning your dilution experimenting with just a few oils. If you buy too many different oils to start, it is very likely you won't be able to use all of them before they deteriorate. As you know, pure essential oils can be costly, so use them wisely. Work with one oil at a time, and get to know each well. Once you've experienced results with these first oils, you're ready to buy more and expand your repertoire.

Measuring Dilutions

The measuring system used for essential oils can be confusing. Some books give dilution measurements in milliliters while others measure in fluid ounces. One simple way to be prepared to use either measuring system is to have measuring devices marked in both milliliters and ounces on hand (these can be found at a biological supply house).

It would be nice to be able to stick with one system of measurement, however most people don't have a milliliter measuring device and many companies sell in ounces and others in milliliters. In the United States, most companies sell products by the ounce, although there is a trend toward converting to milliliters so European recipes measured primarily in milliliters are compatible. For the novice, the best way to start is to measure pure essential oils by the drop. Base oils may be measured either in ounces or in milliliters. I have switched to milliliter bottles in my business to try to avoid confusion. Until aromatherapy practices become more standardized worldwide, measuring systems will be very individual. Measuring in teaspoons and tablespoons is an easy system for the home essential oil user to implement. I very seldom use them because I'm usually blending larger quantities.

Dilution measurements are sometimes given in percentages, such as a "1 percent solution." This means that the essential oil constitutes approximately 1 percent of the total liquid amount. Solutions of 1 to 3 percent are most common in mixing essential oils. A 1 percent solution contains approximately

5 drops of essential oil to 4 teaspoons (20 ml) of carrier (or base) oil. Four teaspoons (20 ml) of oil is usually sufficient for a full body massage. A very mild blend can be made from 1 drop pure essential oil to 2 teaspoons (10 ml) carrier oil.

Basic Dilution Formulas

The best way to proceed in developing a dilution is drop by drop. Start with 1 teaspoon to ½ ounce (5 ml to 15 ml) of carrier so that you make small amounts at a time. Here are some tried and true formulas to begin with until you have the time and skill to develop your own.

HAIR CLEANSING RINSE
Carrier: 2 cups (500 ml) cider vinegar
Essential oil: Up to 10 drops of pure essential oils of your choice. (Juniper, rosemary, rose geranium, clary sage, lavender, lemon, patchouli, or sandalwood work well.)
Dilute: 1 tablespoon (15 ml) of vinegar/essential oil mixture in 2 cups (500 ml) of water.
Use: Rinse through wet hair after shampooing to rid hair of residue build-up. Vinegar rinses may be drying if used everyday, so it is best to restrict their use to two times a week.

HAIR CONDITIONER
Carrier: 1 teaspoon (5 ml) store-bought conditioner of your choice plus 1 teaspoon (5 ml) cider vinegar
Essential oil: 1 drop patchouli and 2 drops rose geranium
Dilution: 2 cups (500 ml) warm water
Use: Rinse diluted mixture through freshly washed hair and rinse. This leaves hair tangle-free, shiny, and smelling earthy and fresh. After rinsing with this mixture and putting my damp hair up while I work, I enjoy letting it down in the evening and brushing out the sweet smell. Try using other essential oil combinations as well.

SHAMPOO
Carrier: One 12–15-ounce bottle of shampoo (unscented is preferable)

Essential oil: 10–15 drops of clary sage, jasmine absolute, juniper, lemon, lavender, rosemary, rosewood, or sandalwood oils, or any combination of these oils.

The following formulas can be made with carrier and essential oils of your choice.

AROMATHERAPY BATH
Carrier: Tub of warm water
Essential oil: 6 to 8 drops
Use: Add oils just prior to entering the tub and mix well. Dilute with ¼ cup milk or cream, or 1 tablespoon carrier oil, if desired.

CARPET FRESHENER
Carrier: 2 cups (500 ml) pure borax
Essential oil: Up to 25 drops
Use: Mix well. Test for staining before applying to large area.

DISHWASHING FORMULA
Carrier: Sink full of dishwashing water and soap
Essential oil: 6 to 10 drops

FACIAL OIL
Carrier: ½ ounce (15 ml) carrier oil
Essential oil: 6 drops
Use: Apply 5 drops of the blend to the face every other night for two weeks.

FRAGRANT BODY LOTION
Carrier: 8-ounce bottle of plain unscented non-mineral-oil-based lotion
Essential oil: 20 to 30 drops (no cinnamon oil)

FRAGRANT BATH SALTS
Carrier: 2 cups (500 ml) sea salt
Essential oil: 10 to 15 drops (no cinnamon oil)

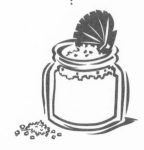

HAND AND SHOWER LIQUID SOAP
Carrier: 4 ounces (118 ml) liquid castile soap

Essential oil: 15 to 25 drops
Use: This soap works great on a loofah sponge, and can help deter the bacteria that builds up on loofah when left damp. Also works well on a small nail brush.

HOUSE CLEANING WATER
Carrier: 2 gallons (8 litres) warm water
Essential Oil: 10 to 25 drops (I like to add Murphy's oil soap to the water as well, according to the manufacturer's directions and depending on the difficulty of the cleaning job.)

INSECT REPELLENT SPRAY
Carrier: 4 ounces (118 ml) water in spray bottle
Essential oil: 5 to 10 drops
Use: Shake as you spray. Don't spray around face and eyes.

MASSAGE, BATH, OR BODY OIL
Carrier: 2 ounces (60 ml) carrier oil
Essential oil: 25 drops (reduce proportionally to make smaller batches)

PERSONAL PERFUME
Carrier: ½ ounce (15 ml) alcohol or jojoba oil
Essential oil: 10 to 15 drops

ROOM FRESHENER
Carrier: 16 ounces (500 ml) water in spray bottle
Essential oil: 20 to 30 drops
Use: Spritz this on furniture, drapes, carpets, and car interior. I also spray this around the damp shower to deter mildew growth. It smells better than most commercial products.

ROOM FRESHENER/INHALER
Carrier: Water in simmer pot
Essential oil: 6 to 10 drops

HERBAL HAIR RINSES

These rinses are made from the herbs themselves, not the essential oils. Essential oils may be added to these blends by the drop, but the proportions here refer to dried herbs in the cut and sifted form.

To make: Combine equal parts of the herbs in the selected combination (see following). Start with 1 tablespoon of each herb and see how you like the result. You can increase the amount later and store the blend, if desired. I usually store dried blends in dark glass jars. Fresh herbs may also be used, but you must increase the amount by three times to get the same potency as dried herbs. The essential oils are concentrated in the dried herbs and less is needed to achieve the same effect.

In a non-metal pan, bring 2 cups of water to a boil. Add 6–10 tablespoons of herb mixture. Turn off heat and cover pan tightly for 20 minutes. Strain herb mixture, cool, and use as a final rinse for the hair. This rinse can be rinsed out after five minutes or left on longer, if desired.

Herb combinations. *For light hair:* chamomile flowers, Calendula petals, nettle*, comfrey, and lemon peel or juice. *For dark hair:* rosemary, nettle, horsetail, red clover, and garden sage.

*Caution: If you are gathering fresh nettle, wear good gloves and be aware that it can cause a nasty rash. Jewel weed, which usually grows nearby, can counteract the effects of a nettle rash. I prefer to use dried nettle. It stimulates hair growth quite nicely.

Variations: Include peppermint, spearmint, rose petals, lemongrass, scented geraniums, basil, lavender, lemon verbena, or lemon balm. The hair rinse combinations can also be added in either fresh or dried form to 2 cups of cider vinegar. Use 2 teaspoons of the herbal vinegar added to 2 cups water for a final rinse.

PERSONAL PERFUMES

Perfume has intrigued man, and surely woman, for centuries. The word perfume is from the Latin *per* (through) and *fumum* (smoke or by fire), referring to the fact that perfumes were originally incense-type mixtures that were offered up to the gods to sweeten one's prayers. Deriving pleasure from scents is an ancient practice and crosses almost every culture. Originally, perfumes were concocted from natural ingredients.

Most modern perfumes, however, are made primarily of synthetic aromatic chemicals. These aromatic chemicals do not have the power to move us the way pure essential oil blends do. The components of anything applied to the body is absorbed by it. This in itself should make us cautious about what we use. I believe the advent of synthetic aromatic chemicals was in response to popular demand for consistency, price control, and supply. Manufacturers couldn't rely upon the graces of nature for producing mass quantities of their products inexpensively. The Chinese believed that every perfume is a medicine. I am sure this refers to natural perfumes, and hints at aromatherapy.

A detailed and entertaining history of perfumes, including the bottles, can be found in a wonderful book entitled, *Fragrance, The Story of Perfume from Cleopatra to Chanel,* by Edwin T. Morris. The intriguing story this book weaves assures us that pure essential oils have played an important role in human life since the beginning of time, right up to today. People from every walk of life share one common thread: We like good smells and dislike bad ones. It's that simple.

I have been stopped in public on several occasions and asked by a passer-by, "What is that marvelous scent you are wearing?" This question often comes from a gentleman who is inquiring how to acquire this scent for his wife or loved one. At that point, I have to stop and take personal inventory to figure out what they are smelling. I may have been bottling pure essential oils that day, or working with some other herbal and aromatic substances that may have clung to my clothing. On other occasions the passer-by may be experiencing one of my homemade perfumes that I put together just for me.

Natural perfume-making is fun to do, and the rewards are wonderful, aromatic substances that enhance the quality of life, instead of synthetic aromatic chemicals that often fade out to somewhat less of a scent than one had hoped for. It can also be economical. Often most of the price you're paying for a commercial perfume is for the bottle, packaging, and promotion of the product.

Assessing Your Scent Likes and Dislikes

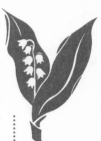

I recall having a keen interest in perfumes early in my life. My first true love once asked me which perfume I would like for Christmas. I gave him a long list, hoping to acquire a few to test on him. Much to my delight, he presented me with bottles of all those I had listed. I felt like a queen, having all of those fragrances with which to surround myself. This experience instilled in me a love of aromatic substances that will last a lifetime.

Throughout the years, very few perfumes have held my interest. They always seemed to lack depth and staying power. I don't like smelling like everyone else, although the perfume ads promised you won't. Each person's own personal chemistry interacts with the scents we wear in various ways. I have often wondered just exactly why and how we choose a certain scent. I conduct a workshop called, "Own Your Own Aroma," in which we explore just that. I ask the participants to consider these questions:

- How did you choose the perfume or fragrance you wear?
- Is it one you chose or did your husband, wife, or lover choose it for you?
- What exactly do you like about that scent? What would you change if you could?
- What are your scent preferences? Do herbal, woodsy, floral, citrus, earthy, or fruity scents appeal to you the most?
- Where do you apply your perfume? Does it last as long as you would like it to?
- Did you buy it for its fragrance or does that pretty bottle just look nice on your dressing table?
- Do you prefer different scents for the changing seasons? Do your scent moods change with your emotional ones?

- Do you have a number of scents or are you loyal to a particular one?
- Would you like the idea of your personal perfume to help reduce stress or enhance your attractiveness?
- How would you like to be able to blend other personal care products to match your preferred scents?
- Do you prefer an alcohol or oil base?

These questions are a good starting point for natural, personal perfume-making.

SUPPLIES FOR PERFUME-MAKING

For making natural perfumes, you will need a variety of pure essential oils, alcohols, and base oils, eyedroppers, bottles, a notepad and pencil, and labels.

Essential Oils

Perfume-making requires a variety of types, or "notes" of essential oils — including top, middle, and base notes. These terms used for the blending of perfumes correspond to the creation of music, since you're creating "a fragrance symphony," so to speak. The classification of these notes varies depending on who is listing them. The listing here is meant to be just a simple guide line. For a more detailed analysis, refer to Robert Tisserand's, *The Art of Aromatherapy,* which has charts listing notes, odor intensity, evaporation rates, and a volatility index.

You do not need to stick to any hard, fast rules to create a perfume. However, a working knowledge of pure essential oils and their individual scents is helpful. I started blending perfumes by adding essential oils to already existing perfumes to enhance their fragrance. Although this was not a true natural perfume, it was a beginning.

Top notes. These are the scents you notice first. They are sharp, but they do not last very long. Moreover, these essential oils account for a small percentage of the final blend. Top notes include: bergamot, lemon, orange, peppermint, chamomile, lime, lemongrass.

Middle notes. These are added to smooth out a blend. These usually form the body of a blend and are used in a higher concentration. Middle notes include: rosewood, lavender, rose geranium, ylang-ylang.

Base notes. These oils add fullness to a blend — the scent that lasts longest. They are deep and earthy scents. These oils are often referred to as fixatives, as they tend to fix the scent and make it last longer on the skin although they account for a very small proportion of the blend. Base notes include: patchouli, sandalwood, vetiver, frankincense, myrrh, and labdanum.

In general, citrus oils lend a fruity note, spice oils a spicy one, and florals can sweeten a blend. The herbal oils add a green note and the root oils deepen a blend. For formula ideas on developing more sensuous blends, consult a fun little book that I picked up in England entitled, *Aromatics* by Valerie Ann Worwood. It includes drop-by-drop recipes and some interesting information that few other publications address.

The possibilities are limited only by your imagination and, of course, your budget!

Blending Perfumes

There are many references on blending in some of the aromatherapy publications listed in the Resources. The scents one likes play an important part in knowing where to start in blending a personal perfume. Experimentation is the best way to experience the scents that can be created. Blend one drop at a time. You can always add more, but you can't remove an oil, and may ruin a blend trying to cover up a mistake. Oils such as ylang-ylang are very odor intense and can overpower a blend.

There are a few different methods for blending. Some people prefer to blend the pure essential oils together first, and then add them to the base. Others prefer to add essential oils to the base drop by drop, testing the blend as they go. Choose the method that works best for you.

Be sure to keep track of your recipes and be brave enough to try variations on them. How do you think Coco Chanel got to Chanel No. 5? I would guess that she had to go through numbers 1–4 first. Naming your perfume blends can be fun. Many a celebrity has lent their name to a fragrance, so why shouldn't you? Be creative and, most of all, have fun!

Selecting a Base

There are several bases you can use for perfume-making, depending on if you like a liquid or oil base. I prefer an oil base on my skin, but make an alcohol-base scent to spray on my clothes and in my hair. Natural perfumemakers debate what is the best alcohol base. I prefer to use Evercleer, a pure grain alcohol (95 percent alcohol, or 190 proof). It is unavailable in some states, however. Vodka is the next best thing.

I often make spice or vanilla alcohol to add to my perfumes. To do this, simply add a whole vanilla bean or 2 tablespoons of spices (allspice, cloves, cinnamon, star anise, and ginger) to a pint of Evercleer or Vodka. Let this mixture sit for 4 weeks. The resulting alcohol lends a warm spicy note to a perfume. It is similar to an herbal tincture in that the alcohol extracts the scent from the vanilla or spices just as it extracts the healing substances in herbs.

You could simply add the pure essential oils of spices directly to the alcohol. I find the scented alcohol more subtle in fragrance, and prefer it over the pure essential oils that can be so overpowering. If you choose to use the pure essential oils, please use caution as some of the spice oils such as clove and cinnamon can be irritating to sensitive skin.

If you choose an oil base, jojoba oil is a good choice. Jojoba is actually a liquid wax that doesn't go rancid as quickly as some of the other base oils. It is kind to the skin and hair. It applies nicely to the skin and tends to last longer.

Bottling

Pretty perfume bottles are enjoying a comeback and you will probably be able to find a nice selection. I have a little 1-ounce cut-glass bottle a young lady gave me one year for Christmas. It was very inexpensive and I have gotten a lot of use from it. Bottles with a bulb-type top are perfect for alcohol-base perfumes. For oil-base ones, stick to the dark glass bottles that you use for other blends such as massage oils and nail oils. A 4 ml dropper top bottle is perfect.

A personal perfume is a most welcome gift — one that says your perfumes should be as unique as your personality. I warn you, though, playing with perfume-making can become addictive and you will never look at (or smell) store-bought perfumes quite the same way ever again. I have made perfumes for teachers, stressed-out executives, busy homemakers, and lively teenagers.

No one has ever complained about an allergy to a natural perfume that I have produced, although I often hear people complain about allergic reactions to synthetic versions. I personally believe the allergic reaction may be caused by the synthetic aromatic chemicals used in the production of perfume, which are avoided with a natural product. Alcohol can be drying to the skin, so only a small amount should be sprayed at a time.

RECIPES FOR PERSONAL PERFUME BLENDS

Remember, each individual has his or her own preferences, and experimentation is the key to finding the oils that suit you best.

I suggest adding the essential oils to the bottle first, then adding the alcohol. I have found that if I add more oils after I have added the alcohol, the blend may become cloudy. If this doesn't matter to you, blend away.

If you don't use the scented alcohol, then 1–2 drops of the preferred essential oil may be added. For example, when making the CKD I blend, I may add 1–2 drops of vanilla oleoresin instead of the scented alcohol.

CKD I
I love to spritz this perfume in my hair.

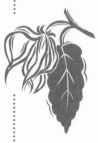

3 drops rose absolute (to give the perfume a rosy, golden color)
3 drops jasmine absolute
5 drops lavender
5 drops sandalwood
2 drops ylang-ylang
1 ounce vanilla alcohol or ½ ounce jojoba oil
(use oil blend directly on skin only)

CHAPTER 13
Other Uses for Essential Oils

Pure essential oils can be of service in a variety of uncommon places. I have used them to enhance every place from airports to musty hotel rooms. Pure essentials have accompanied and assisted me on journeys into difficult situations like visiting hospitals and nursing homes and attending funerals. These oils have made the subways of Paris and London easier to bear on an unusually hot summer day and the streets of the city a little less scary to travel — my confidence and alertness enhanced by jasmine absolute and rosemary. As a personal perfume, essential oils have stimulated interesting conversations with complete strangers and carried thoughts and memories to friends and loved ones far away on aromatic breezes via the postal service.

Pure essential oils heighten my spirits and soothe my soul. They often announce the presence of a visitor before the person is actually seen, and provide fragrant reminders after they have gone. Through all of life's adventures, pure essential oils aid me in assimilating a variety of circumstances. They have the ability to increase beauty, reduce stress, and make a significant contribution to human experience.

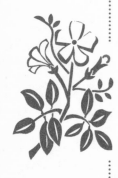

MAKING TRAVEL MORE ENJOYABLE

Traveling can provide an opportunity to experience pure essential oils that you haven't tried before or to use old favorites in new ways. Long hot car rides can create cranky travelers. Carry a jug of water with a few drops of peppermint oil in it to apply to the face, neck, and arms with a washcloth to cool and soothe the weary ones. Lavender essential oil helps travelers to relax on long trips. In the car, carry a spritz bottle of water combined with a few drops of lavender. When traveling by plane, put a few drops on tissues and carry them in a small plastic bag.

Essential oils can enhance the car environment by adding a stimulating or relaxing influence, depending on individual needs. For a nervous driver, lavender may be of assistance. For a weary driver, rest is of the utmost importance, yet rosemary,

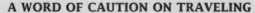

A WORD OF CAUTION ON TRAVELING

If you're traveling by airplane or into other countries and carrying essential oils, be prepared to explain what you have in those little bottles. I once had an airport security person mistake my wooden box of oils for shotgun shells on an x-ray and made me empty out my bags. I also found out the hard way not to stand around in a busy international airport inhaling deeply from little dark glass bottles. Security asked me to come with them and explain exactly what was in that bottle. I have never explained aromatherapy so eloquently or quickly in my life! This experience led me to develop a new product — travel tissues with essential oils that can be carried in a small plastic bag.

Customs officers are probably becoming better informed about essential oils, but don't count on it. Duty can also be confusing when importing large amounts of pure essential oils. I tried importing large amounts from England years ago and it was a nightmare. I'm sure it has become easier now, however, I only order small amounts from abroad and stick to domestic suppliers for bulk quantities. Larger companies have staff to deal with this much better than you or I can.

When you ship to or from overseas, make sure your pure essential oils are well packaged. I once received a lovely scented order from England in which all of the rose otto had spilled. I usually wrap each bottle in plastic to ensure that the labels on other bottles in the order won't be ruined by a spill or breakage. This is a great way to reuse and recycle plastic bubble wrap.

peppermint, and/or lemon can help brighten the senses. I put essential oils on a clay pot. After the oils have soaked in, I put it under the seat of my car.

I also create dash bags — combinations of herbs and oils that can be placed on the car dashboard and, with the heat turned on high, allowed to diffuse the scent. My friend Mary Lou used her Sniffy Bag™ (see recipe on page 135) when she had a cold but had to travel. Her truck became a sauna filled with redolent vapors that helped her breathe easier. After using it this way, she applied some sniffy bag refresher oil to revive the scent of her sniffy bag.

Air travel presents a number of challenges to the body. Take along a bottle of homemade rosewater to hydrate the skin and soothe the spirit. It also helps to drink plenty of water and eat lightly. Adding a squeeze of fresh lemon to your water can be refreshing. I have found that asking for a vegetarian meal on a flight, although I'm not a strict vegetarian, often gets me a meal that is a little more palatable. Drinking herb teas instead of soda or alcoholic drinks helps you stay balanced. I bring along my own tea bags and simply ask for hot water.

Jet lag can be eased somewhat by the use of pure essential oils. Acupuncture tacks put in the ears can also be helpful, by stimulating certain points in the body that are linked to alertness and balance. I did this once when I had only one week to be in England. Some people noticed what they may have thought of as my "new age" earrings and gave me puzzled looks, but the tacks did the job.

A massage before leaving and upon arriving at your destination can ease a long journey, especially when suffering from what I call "luggage shoulders." When a massage isn't available try a warm bath with lavender, geranium, chamomile, peppermint, or grapefruit oil. Grapefruit and peppermint are good pick-me-ups, while lavender, geranium, and chamomile are relaxing.

Pure essential oils are also useful in making yourself at home in an anonymous hotel room. One of the first things I do upon entering a hotel room is fill the sink with hot water and some of my favorite essential oils. I also wipe down the bed and spray some of my homemade perfume upon the pillows. These familiar scents immediately make me feel more at ease. Friends at herbal conferences are often able to "sniff out" my hotel room by following the vapors emitting from under the door of my room into the hallway.

CREATING A WELCOMING, CONDUCIVE WORK ENVIRONMENT

The way a place of business smells greatly affects the reactions employees, customers, and visitors have to the establishment. Think about it: When you enter a very nice-looking pub that smells of stale smoke and old beer, you don't feel much like staying to enjoy a meal. Grocery stores with the scent of rotting food aren't conducive to welcoming shoppers. I have been asked to do aromatherapy sessions in salons that reek of nail and hair chemicals, but I can't work in such a harshly scented environment.

When someone enters your place of business their first impression is made with their nose — a fact that most businesses don't realize. Think about the hours you've spent sitting in stale-smelling waiting rooms of doctors, lawyers, and city offices, and how they've made you feel. Then think about the enticing aromas of a coffee shop — even people who don't like the taste of coffee often say they love being around the smell of it. Or the toasty warm spicy scents that envelop you when you walk into a bakery, making you hungry for a goodie. It's no coincidence that the cinnamon roll shop at the mall is often close to the entrance — welcoming consumers. Even the astronauts on the space shuttle noted that the lemon-scented hand wipes they used enhanced the rather bland environment inside the shuttle. Movie theaters have known for years that blowing around that popcorn smell makes you want to indulge!

Use Inviting Scents

I know a chiropractor who scents his office with sweet orange oil. Sitting in his waiting room is much more pleasurable than the usual waiting rooms. Good magazines aren't enough to keep folks from becoming impatient. Olfactory stimulation can help people feel much differently about waiting for or even going to an appointment. Many people hate the smells associated with going to the dentist almost as much as the sound of the drill. What if the dentist used an aromatic diffuser to enhance the treatment room with the scents of lemon or lavender?

Perhaps a blend could be designed for the specific office, based on a scent survey of patients' preferences. The scent of almost any pure essential oil is preferable to the smell of bad or drilled teeth! The oils may also have the effect of helping the patient to relax during a procedure, especially if the patient were given the blend in advance with advice to smell it at relaxing times, thus developing an association between the scent and relaxation.

Selecting the scent for a business is largely a matter of personal choice. I've often heard it said that since all people don't like the same scent, it is better to use nothing. But you can do your own research to discover what your employees and clients like. You will always have a few folks who object to a certain scent no matter what you choose, but it will surely enhance a visit for the majority of clients and customers. I had a work-study student who was the nurse at my gynecologist's office. When I went in to the office under stressful conditions contemplating surgery (which I never end up having), she gave me a piece of gauze with chamomile, neroli (orange blossom), and lavender on it prior to seeing the doctor. This was an act of kindness that certainly made my visit easier to bear.

Real estate agents call me often to request scents to use in homes they are selling. Vanilla wins hands-down when it comes to scenting a home. People have actually called to tell me they bought the house because it smelled so good, and could I please make them up some more of the scent they love!

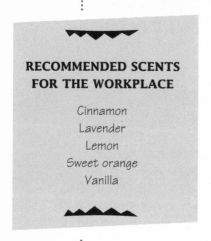

RECOMMENDED SCENTS FOR THE WORKPLACE

Cinnamon
Lavender
Lemon
Sweet orange
Vanilla

Introducing the Scent

Workplace scent can be diffused in a number of ways. Aromatic diffusers work wonders in changing a building's scent. These are now available with built-in timers that go on and off as needed. Carpet freshener made from borax and pure essential oils can be used by the cleaning staff. Tissues with a drop or two of pure essential oils or a blend can be given to individual patients or clients. One of my massage therapists uses a spray of pure essential oils to wipe down her massage table between clients.

We've just begun to explore the many ways essential oils could be used to enhance public environments. Schools all seem to have their own unique and memorable scents. Could school children learn or behave better in a room scented with essential oils? I have already had a number of teachers come to me for help in doing just this.

I have often wondered how essential oils might be used to alter the environment in prisons. Research has been done on the effects of various paint colors on aggressive behavior. Could scent also be used to improve behavior in a contained environment? Perhaps it could help in facilities for the mentally ill, as well.

Japanese researchers are exploring the possibilities of increasing productivity and reducing error by pumping essential oil of lemon into an office building. While this raises important issues about manipulation in the workplace, it also acknowledges the potential effects essential oils may have.

Think about the offensive workplace smells that could be improved by the use of essential oils. The scent of a synthetically treated public restroom is nauseating and overpowering. The unpleasant odor often lingers in your nose long afterwards. The scent of an elevator crowded with people wearing synthetic perfumes and colognes can be an olfactory nightmare. Some offices and public meeting places are actually banning the use of perfumes. The subways I have ridden on in the world could surely use some aromatherapy! Buses and taxis could as well. Gyms and locker rooms definitely could use pure essential oils.

Take notice the next time you enter a building. How does it smell? Does this scent affect how you feel about that business? Then think about how your own place of business smells. Consider ways in which you might use essential oils to make it a more inviting, enjoyable place in which to work and spend time.

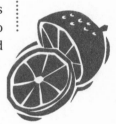

CARING FOR THE ELDERLY AND SICK

Pure essential oils can be valuable in improving the daily living of senior citizens. While the sense of smell does diminish somewhat in the elder years, the capacity to enjoy fresh scents (unless the sense of smell is entirely gone) never does. Bringing essential oils into the home are a way of stimulating memories and pleasant feelings for people who can't get out as much as they did when they were younger.

Ask an elder in your life what scents they have loved throughout their lives, and think of ways of incorporating these essential oils into their lives. I love speaking to senior citizen groups. They always have entertaining stories and aromatic memories to share that stay with me long after the visit is over.

One wonderful way for elders to enjoy essential oils is a refreshing basin bath. This is quick and easy to prepare. Just add 1 or 2 drops of lavender, rose geranium, bergamot, frankincense, rosewood, or sandalwood (or other oils of choice) to a basin of water and wash the skin with a washcloth. Follow up with a non-mineral oil moisture cream or a base oil with the same essential oils to condition the skin.

In the Hospital

Pure essential oils can truly help to ease the suffering, and improve the environment, for anyone enduring a hospital stay. The sense of smell can often be of service to our souls when other parts of our body, mind, and spirit have tired.

When my long-time friend Frank was dying due to complications of diabetes, his loved ones filled his last days in the hospital and at home with hospice care with supportive people and pure essential oils. We massaged him with melissa, lavender, rose otto, patchouli, and grapefruit. He enjoyed sandalwood massaged into his feet, and dearly loved lavender rubbed into his beard. Being totally blind, Frank found the scents much more intense, and he was able to enjoy the fragrances fully. As I worked with him people would stop and poke their head in his room and ask, "What smells so good in here?" I call that the olfactory hook — it reaches out into the environment and invites one to enjoy the bounty of nature.

Before using oils in the hospital, be sure to check first with other patients in the room to make sure that the scents won't disturb them in any way. If others object, ask for your friend to be moved to a room where you can use them. In the hospital, I usually keep massage confined to hands and feet, depending on the patient's condition. When treating someone who is sick, it is particularly important to keep your blends on the light side. Remember: Less is best.

It is my hope that one day pure essential oil will help in hospitals, nursing homes, hospices, funeral homes, and many more of those places that somehow linger in our minds and are often associated with negative emotions. Along with the antibacterial powers many essential oils have, they could perhaps make some of life's transitions a bit easier to bear.

In a Nursing Home

While acting as guardian to a wonderful woman named Mildred Bowren, I found out just how useful essential oils could be in easing pain and promoting comfort. "Ma" Bowren, as I always called her, had led a full life. She was foster parent to over 300 children in her career and ran a working farm at the same time. She and Frank Bowren were hard-working folks that probably never gave their sense of smell a lot of thought unless the lilacs were blooming or the smokehouse was full. Mildred came into my care after Frank died. I was one of the few young charges that ever sought her out in adulthood.

Mildred moved into a small apartment for a few years, but it eventually became necessary to admit her to a nursing home due to her health. Many people have negative reactions to the scent of nursing homes and hospitals. I decided to make Mildred's stay as pleasant as possible through the use of pure essential oils.

I started out by bringing home her laundry. Although the nursing home offers laundry service, her clothes could be line-dried and lightly scented with lavender for a calming influence as well as a familiar one. I had watched Mildred hang out laundry many times so I knew the scent of line-dried clothes was comforting to her. The association between freshly laundered clothes and lavenders dates back centuries when bed linens were hung upon lavender hedges to dry in the sun. When I hung her clothes in her closet they retained their fresh scent for days.

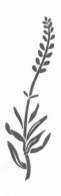

I also made lavender sachets to tuck in her dresser drawer (and asked a willing nurse to squeeze it every time she got something out of the drawer for Mildred), and stick it in the corner of her pillowcase at night. People have enjoyed the pleasant scent and relaxing effects of lavender sachets for centuries. This is another custom worthy of reviving.

Another custom I have always enjoyed, as did Mildred, is using rosemary in the hair — in herbal hair rinses, vinegars, and conditioning essential oil blends. Rosemary has enjoyed a rich history in helping keep the hair glossy and the mind bright.

Rosemary has traditionally signified remembrance. "There's rosemary that's for remembrance. Pray, you love, remember," wrote William Shakespeare. It was a treat for

MAKING A LAVENDER SACHET

Materials Needed:
A handful of lavender flowers
An 8" x 10" piece of cloth (finely woven lace is nice, so you can
see the lavender but it doesn't fall out when squeezed)
A small rubber band
A 12" piece of ribbon

I call this my "no sew, basic, easy-on-the-herbalist" sachet. In other words, it's very easy to complete and a great task when you need to relax. Make several at a time so you will have them on hand as a welcome gift for a friend or loved one under stress. An occasional squeeze will freshen this sachet by releasing the essential oils contained in the little flower buds. These sachets last for years.

To make: Cut the cloth rectangle. Pile a handful of lavender into the center of the cloth (see Figure 1). Wrap up the sides and join tightly with the rubber band (see Figure 2). Tie a ribbon bow over the rubber band (see Figure 3).

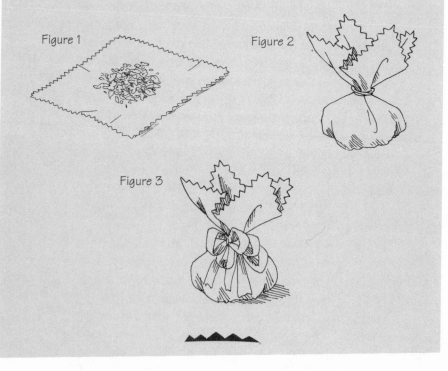

Figure 1

Figure 2

Figure 3

Mildred to have her hair done with a brush sprinkled with rosemary oil, and she always remembered it enough to ask for it again and again, although she was considered to be in the early stages of Alzheimer's disease. Research is underway in England on how rosemary essential oil can aid those with Alzheimer's retain and access their memories.

A pomander always hung in Mildred's closet to give off the spicy aroma of cinnamon and cloves. I wiped down her bed and bathroom with oils such as rosemary, lavender, rose geranium, and eucalyptus. I would add 20 drops of pure essential oils to a 16-ounce (500 ml) spray bottle and often sprayed the curtains, her mattress, and bathroom.

When I asked the nursing staff why pure essential oils — which are antiseptic, antiviral, and antibacterial — were not employed more by institutions, I was told that would be masking odors. When I tried to explain that herbs were burned in hospitals for centuries to clear the air, and how powerful an oil like thyme which contains thymol can be in keeping us safe from contagion, my words fell upon deaf ears, although their noses appreciated my efforts.

Additional things like peeling a fresh orange by her bed and sharing it with her gave her great pleasure, and massages on her arthritic hands and legs were met with deep sighs of satisfaction whenever she began to feel the effects of the lavender, rosemary, and juniper in almond oil that I used.

Mildred's whole sense of being would change after these times together. I know the quality of her stay was greatly enhanced by the use of pure essential oils in her room. I also think the nurses were so attentive, in part, because of how comfortable her room felt with its sweetly scented contents.

CARING FOR PETS

New information is emerging on pets and aromatherapy massage. One must heed even a bit more caution then when using pure essential oils on humans. For one thing, animal skin absorbs oils at a different rate than human skin. (For more on this, see *The Essential Oil Safety Data Manual* by Robert Tisserand.)

Essential oils that have been found helpful in working with animals to confront everything from flea control to depression include: lavender, tea tree, chamomile, bergamot, cedarwood, juniper, rosemary, sandalwood, geranium, patchouli, sweet orange, and eucalyptus. The one essential oil you should *avoid* using on pets is pennyroyal. This popular flea repellant is much too concentrated in pure essential oil form.

Flea and Tick Control

Dried herbs and essential oils can be very effective in shielding your animal from fleas and ticks. See my recipe for pet powder on page 139. Keep pets out of the room while the powder is being applied and absorbed. I have seen a full-blown tick drop off of a dog onto the floor when a single drop of undiluted tea tree oil was applied directly. Cleaning pet bedding with pure essential oils helps repel vermin.

You can make an herbal bug-repellant pillow for a cat or dog by adding equal amounts of lavender flowers, cedarwood chips and pennyroyal herb *(not oil)* to the stuffing of a pillow or small homemade pet bed mattress. If you're substituting pure essential oils for the dried herbs, use only 5 drops total per pillow or mattress and, again, avoid pennyroyal oil. I know it is listed in many pet recipes, but I feel it is much too strong to be used directly on an animal. Also avoid using irritating citrus oils. While they are an ingredient in many flea repellants, they are used highly diluted. I once witnessed a small kitten go into convulsions after an unsuspecting owner applied orange oil to its fur. I would not suggest using pure essential oils with young puppies or kittens. I tend to use homeopathy with my cats and they very seldom have the need for pure essential oils.

Pure essential oils may, however, be added in small amounts to a pet's bathwater, approximately 8 drops of essential oil to two gallons of water. Eucalyptus, lavender, juniper, cedarwood, peppermint, or tea tree work well.

> ▼▼▼▼▼
> **CAUTION**
>
> Always consult a qualified veterinarian before attempting to treat a pet's potentially serious condition on your own.
> ▲▲▲▲▲

Other Pet Health Care Treatments

One solution I have found effective in helping to clear up minor cuts, scrapes, and other little irritations for both pets and humans is a tincture of myrrh. This is a highly astringent product, and it helped heal a very nasty abscess on my cat Buddy's side when he received a puncture wound from another cat. I diluted 1 dram (4 ml) of the myrrh tincture into 2 cups of warm water and applied compresses of this every hour until the wound was completely drained. I then applied tincture of myrrh undiluted to close and heal the wound and the place the doctor had lanced it to enable it to drain. I didn't apply the tincture undiluted at first, to enable the wound to drain before it closed up.

When Buddy had a problem with his skin, due to feline diabetes, I applied pure essential oils and herbal salves which were quite effective. I started by applying a 10 percent mixture of lavender, tea tree, geranium, and patchouli in sweet almond oil. I used this combination of oils first to eliminate any possible parasite problem and condition the skin. Buddy didn't take too well to the strong scent, and retaliated by taking a nap in his litter box. I then applied a 2 percent dilution of the same essential oil mixture in sweet almond oil for three days, twice a day.

FORMULA FOR TINCTURE OF MYRRH

Combine 1 ounce myrrh gum with 4 ounces 90 or more proof alcohol (I prefer Evercleer or vodka) in an airtight glass jar. Let stand for two weeks before using.

This formula has been effective for treating both me and my cat, Buddy. Personally, I use myrrh tincture to clear up a cold sore almost instantly or to drain and heal an unsightly pimple as quick as possible. I carry a 4 ml bottle with me when I travel. I have also employed astringent, antiseptic myrrh to a badly bleeding cut, and witnessed its effectiveness at stopping the bleeding. And Buddy can surely vouch for myrrh tincture's effectiveness at treating his abcesses!

Following the oil treatment, I began a massage routine on Buddy's scaly, cracked skin with undiluted sandalwood oil (3 to 5 drops massaged into his head three times a day). This was costly and truly worth it — and having Buddy smell of sandalwood was quite pleasant for him and for me! All of the bad skin came off, leaving bald spots, and the skin began to heal quite

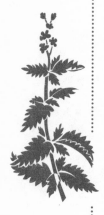

nicely. I switched over to an herbal salve with comfrey in it for the last two weeks and Buddy's head healed beautifully.

Buddy also seemed to enjoy licking the salve off his paws. Remember that most animals will lick off whatever you apply if they can reach the spot. For this reason, you should use caution about what you apply because animals react differently to certain substances than humans do. When I used peroxide to clean out and aerate Buddy's abscess he didn't appreciate the fuzzy feel of it on his tongue one bit. In contrast, the herbal salves he licked off were made from fresh herbs, a much less concentrated form of plant material than pure essential oils.

Buddy has returned to his old self. He hisses at Rosemary, our other kitty, just as he had done before he got sick, and showed a return of his routine spirit. I can judge his state of health by whether or not he comes to bed. When he became sick he wouldn't leave the food or water dish. Now he has returned to keep me warm at night. He is playful, active, loves his catnip bag again, is gaining weight, cleaning himself very nicely, and is very affectionate.

PART III:
HERBAL BODY CARE

▼▼▼

Naturally Refreshing Wraps,
Rubs, Lotions, Masks,
Oils, and Scrubs

Greta Breedlove

CHAPTER 14

Making and Enjoying Spa Treatments

There are a lot of good reasons to make your own skin-care products. Many people are opting for a natural approach to lifestyle, from dietary choices to skin-care products. By making your own treatments, you can be sure of exactly what goes into them. Some of you, like me, may have experienced allergic reactions to many commercial skin-care products and seek natural products out of necessity. Maybe you feel that commercial skin-care products are too expensive. There are many treatments that you can do for yourself at home for a fraction of the cost of a salon visit.

HEAD-TO-TOE TREATMENTS

Beginning with the head and face and working our way down the body with treatments for the full torso, the hands, and finally the feet, you'll find pampering here for every part of the body. I also encourage you to share these relaxing treatments with friends and loved ones.

Before introducing you to the ingredients, supplies, and simple equipment you'll need, I would like to encourage you to think about the ideas in this book as part of a larger whole — your health and well-being. Radiant, healthy skin is a result of many factors: a healthy diet, plenty of exercise, good skin-care practices, and a positive, relaxed mental attitude.

ADOPTING A LIFESTYLE FOR RADIANT SKIN

A healthy diet is essential to radiant skin. There is so much information available on diets to keep you healthy that I cannot even begin to scratch the surface in this book. However, I will stress that you need to consume plenty of fresh fruits and vegetables every day. (No, potato chips do not qualify as a vegetable!) If you don't like fruits and vegetables, experiment with preparing them in various ways until you find some that you enjoy. Eating a balanced and varied diet is important.

Drink Plenty of Water

Water is crucial for healthy skin, helping to keep it soft and supple. Many of the recipes in this book use water to cleanse the skin externally; but it is even more beneficial when consumed internally. Doctors recommend drinking eight 8-ounce glasses of water each day, and more if you are sick or out in the sun or heat. You will get much better results from your skin-care products and treatments if you consume the recommended amounts of water. One of the side benefits of drinking plenty of water is that it is also helpful if you are trying to lose weight.

Nourish Your Skin with Herbal Teas

Another way to help hydrate the skin and receive vitamins and minerals important to overall health is by drinking herbal teas. They are easy to make and there are any number of different teas to choose from. I like to purchase the loose herbs for making teas (often available in bulk at natural and specialty food stores) rather than tea bags because I can better judge the freshness of the herbs. If you don't have a choice, tea from tea bags is still a good, healthy alternative to soft drinks. Do some tea tasting to see which herbs you like best, and try combining several. If you find a commercial tea-bag combination you like, look at the list of ingredients and try creating your own version. While almost any herbs are good for you, I've listed a few that are particularly nourishing for the skin and hair.

Mixing herbal tea with fruit juice is a great way to get natural sweetness and the benefits of the herbs at the same time. If you are making a juice from concentrate, try using herbal tea in place of the water portion. I usually like to add a little more water as well, because most commercial juices are too sweet for me.

HERBS FOR SKIN AND HAIR

- Black alder (for skin eruptions)
- Bergamot tea (cleanses the system)
- Burdock
- Dandelion
- Horsetail
- Nettles
- Oat straw
- Sarsaparilla
- Stevia
- Yellow dock

MAKING SPA TREATMENTS

Making your own body-care products is easy, fun, nurturing, and liberating. Read this chapter carefully before you dive into the specific recipes in subsequent chapters, so you can establish your work area, have the right equipment on hand, and get your home spa set up for maximum enjoyment.

ASSEMBLING THE EQUIPMENT

To get started making your own herbal body-care products you need look no further than your kitchen for the basic equipment; no special equipment or great cooking skills are required to create the recipes in this book. All you'll need are some common kitchen appliances and equipment and a desire to create.

It is best to reserve the equipment you use for making herbal products solely for this purpose, especially any plastic tools such as spatulas and blenders; glass equipment is easier to clean and sterilize. Some of the essential oils used in many of the recipes may leave a residue that is better left out of your meals. The equipment doesn't have to be new when you start, but once you've used it for this purpose, I don't recommend using it for food preparation. Following are the pieces of equipment you will need.

BLENDER
Used for making moisturizing creams and lotions. Also may be used to grind herbs and grains loosely or to a fine powder. A glass blender is far easier to clean than is the plastic variety.

CUTTING BOARD
It is nice to have several boards of different sizes that can be moved around as needed. I prefer those made of wood, which can be replaced when they become too worn. If you use your cutting board for both meat and herbal products, use plastic cutting boards, which are easier to sanitize and maintain than wood.

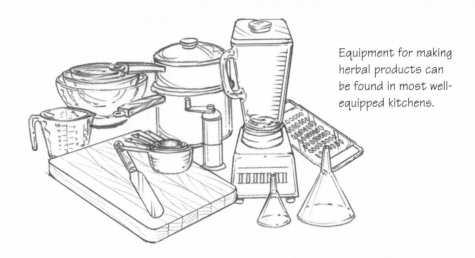

Equipment for making herbal products can be found in most well-equipped kitchens.

DOUBLE BOILER

Produces gentle, even heat, which is especially helpful in making infused herbal oil products such as massage oils, lip balms, eye creams, and moisturizers. It is important that your double boiler be either stainless steel, enamel, or glass. Do not use aluminum, copper, Teflon, or cast iron; these will affect the finished product.

EYEDROPPERS OR PIPETTES

Glass eyedroppers or pipettes are useful for measuring essential oils and resins. These can be purchased through herbal suppliers and bottle and container suppliers.

FUNNELS

You can purchase a set of three sizes of funnels, which will come in handy for filling bottles and containers. I have had a hard time finding widemouthed funnels, but they are easy to make using recycled gallon or half-gallon plastic containers (the kind milk comes in). Simply cut the plastic, maintaining the handle and spout opening. You can also create a scoop/funnel this way.

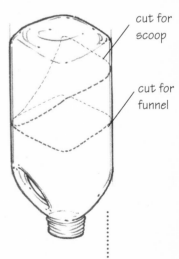

cut for scoop

cut for funnel

GLASS BOWLS

Glass bowls are especially nice to use — and easy to clean — but stainless-steel bowls will also work. You'll need a variety of bowls, from custard size to large mixing bowls.

GLOVES

Dishwashing gloves are okay; however, the closer-fitting latex type allows for fine movements and better dexterity.

GRATER

Useful in grating soap and vegetables. I prefer a plastic grater to the metal one, but either will work. Many books suggest grating beeswax. I usually end up grating my fingers when I attempt this. Instead, I cut the beeswax into small pieces using a paring knife.

MEASURING CUPS AND SPOONS

Helpful in keeping ingredients in proportion to each other. In some recipes, exact measurements can ensure success.

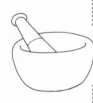

MORTAR AND PESTLE

Great for crushing dried herbs, seeds, flowers, and bark, as well as fresh fruit and vegetable pulps. I recommend the marble variety, although I also have an excellent wooden set.

PARING KNIVES

Great for cutting and chopping herbs, flowers, and fruits; use to sliver beeswax.

SAUCEPANS

Stainless-steel or enamel pans are best. Large spaghetti pots are good for making floral and aromatic waters; smaller pans are also useful.

SPATULA

You can't have too many spatulas. Very useful for scooping and filling containers.

SPICE MILL OR COFFEE GRINDER

A hand-cranked spice mill or coffee grinder is best for grinding oatmeal, almonds, lavender, roses, and any number of other herbs, grains, and seeds. Enjoy the fragrance of the powdered flowers and aromatic herbs. Note: To clean the inner workings of the mill, do not wash or immerse it; simply wipe it clean with a dry cloth. Don't use the same grinder for coffee beans.

STIRRING RODS

Chopsticks, wood or plastic, work well for dispersing scents in oil, but glass chemistry stirring rods are even better and are easier to clean. This is where it pays to have a brother who works in a lab! (Thanks, Larry.) If you're not so lucky, look for laboratory suppliers in the Yellow Pages. Be sure to use new rods that have never been used in toxic chemicals!

STRAINERS

Various meshes and sizes come in very handy, especially in making herbal infusions and grinding nuts. The Vermont Country Store (see Resources) carries a nice set of three at about half the price you'll pay at gourmet cooking shops.

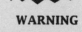

WARNING

Do not use pans and other equipment with copper, aluminum, Teflon, or cast-iron finishes. These materials react with the ingredients in your recipe and will adversely affect the quality of the finished product.

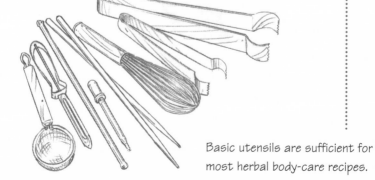

Basic utensils are sufficient for most herbal body-care recipes.

TONGS

The long barbecue type are best for use in body wraps, but the shorter variety will also help protect your hands from hot water.

VEGETABLE PEELER OR ZESTER

Great for removing the zest from citrus fruits and vegetables.

WIRE WHISK

Essential for mixing bath crystals and facial and body scrubs. Helps to distribute the scent throughout these products; besides, it's fun to use.

SELECTING STORAGE CONTAINERS

Bottles and containers can get quite pricey, especially if you make herbal products to give as gifts or to sell. I am always on the lookout for pretty containers. Occasionally, you may find bottles at discount stores, gourmet shops, and gift and specialty stores. I purchase most of my bottles from a local wholesaler, but this requires buying by the case. There are several retail mail-order suppliers that sell containers in smaller quantities (see Resources).

It is helpful to know the common names used to refer to various bottle shapes and styles. Following are descriptions of the ones I use most often.

RECYCLING BOTTLES AND CONTAINERS

When creating products for yourself, recycled containers can be a godsend. Some of my most beautiful containers are finds from flea markets and tag sales. Before you package what you've made, however, be sure to sterilize the container (see page 210). If you are inspired to start your own product line to sell, the FDA requires that you use new containers only.

Glass Containers

Clear glass containers are readily available, but glass in amber and in blue is becoming more popular. These colored glasses better protect products containing oils and dried herbs from light.

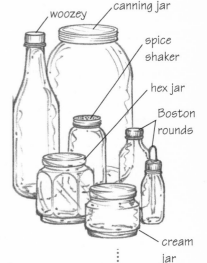

woozey   canning jar

spice shaker

hex jar

Boston rounds

cream jar

CREAM JARS

These pretty jars with wide mouths are excellent for creams and salves.

SPICE SHAKERS

These shakers are usually 2 inches high and are perfect for sprinkling out dried herbs that you might use in small quantities. These containers can be used to dispense your powder preparations because of the shaker tops.

WOOZEYS

These narrow-necked jars are designed for herbal vinegars and wines and come in different sizes. The most common are 5-ounce, 10-ounce, and 12-ounce versions. They can be used for culinary vinegars, bath vinegars, and bath oils.

HEX JARS

These six-sided, widemouthed jars are used by beekeepers for storing honey because of their resemblance to the honeycomb. They are very pretty and useful for creams and moisturizers, although I find the lids to be unreliable for travel.

STORAGE OR CANNING JARS

These jars are usually available in pint, quart, half-gallon, and gallon sizes. I use them to store dried herbs.

BOSTON ROUNDS

These glass jars are available in clear, amber, and cobalt blue. They come in many sizes, from ½ ounce to 16 ounces with either a glass dropper or simply a cap. The colored glass protects products from bright light.

Plastic Containers

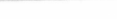

CREAM JARS

These opaque, white, widemouthed jars are great for lip balms, salves, and moisture creams. They are especially convenient for travel.

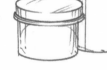

LOTION BOTTLES

Translucent, squeezable, flip-top bottles are perfect for creamy lotions and massage oils.

Other Containers

TINS

Shallow, widemouthed, decorative tins containing a label on the cover are great for salves and lip balms.

POWDER CYLINDERS

These white, lined, cardboard cylinders are excellent containers for herbal body powders and bath crystals. The white cardboard is easy to decorate with stickers or labels.

PRESS-AND-BREW TEA BAGS

These ready-to-make tea bags can be used to create your own tea blends or eye bags. Just place 1 to 2 teaspoons of the herbs in the bag and iron the closure. These are available in several different sizes from herbal suppliers. (See the Resources at the back of the book.)

MUSLIN BAGS

Also available in a variety of sizes, these drawstring bags are useful for making herbal tea (1 cup to 1 gallon) and herbal bath bags.

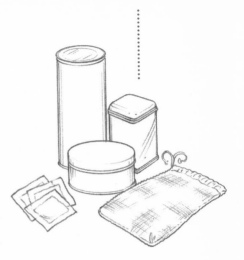

Decorating Containers

This book is full of gift ideas. Since so many of the products you can make are packaged in jars, bottles, tins, or clear plastic bags, stickers are a great way to personalize and decorate your wares. There are many unusual stickers available today, both humorous and beautiful; the search for just the right one for a particular friend can be rewarding and fun.

Find a sticker that illustrates the use for or an ingredient in your product — a hand, a basket of herbs, a bee — or symbolizes something special about your friend — a favorite animal or hobby, for example. Stickers can be found in so many different places: Discount department stores, drugstores, craft stores, stationery stores, and gift shops often carry a variety. Or try your hand at creating your own from blank white labels (available in many different sizes at a stationery store). Children especially like to decorate their own stickers.

Ribbons are an elegant addition to your packaging. Start saving a variety of ribbons and bows. Be sure to recycle any ribbons you receive on gifts. Let your friends know you're collecting, and you may be surprised at the assortment you get from them. If you want to create a down-to-earth look, raffia is just the thing for you. Ribbons and stickers often work well together for that finishing touch.

USING RECYCLED CONTAINERS

Avoid reusing containers that previously held medicine, film, poison, household cleaners, spoiled food, compost, or fertilizer. Use common sense when deciding whether a container is safe to reuse.

Always sterilize any container that has been previously used to ensure the purity of your finished product. If you plan to sell your products, the FDA requires that you use new containers only. Following are the sterilization standards set up by the U.S. Occupational Health and Safety Administration (OSHA).

Sterilizing Glass Containers with Metal Lids

1. Wash the containers and lids thoroughly with soap and water, rinsing several times.
2. Combine ¼ cup bleach with 2 cups of hot water and submerge the clean containers and lids thoroughly in this solution.
3. Fill a large enamel or stainless-steel pot with water.
4. Submerse the bottles and lids, making sure there are no air bubbles left in the bottles.
5. Cover the pot and bring to a rolling boil.
6. Boil for 20 minutes; let cool.
7. Remove bottles and lids from water and allow to air-dry on a sterile towel.

Plastic Containers

Unfortunately, plastic containers are harder to sterilize because the boiling process may melt them. I recommend washing thoroughly and rinsing in the bleach formula; a good dishwashing cycle can also kill many harmful substances that cannot be seen. Use plastic containers to package products that are less prone to spoilage.

Watch for spoilage in your finished products and in the bulk ingredients. Make products in small batches to help reduce the potential for spoilage. If you are concerned about a product or if it smells off, throw it away: Better safe than sorry. If your herbs look old and withered or start to mold, offer them to the compost pile.

CREATING THE SPA EXPERIENCE AT HOME

Setting up a relaxing atmosphere is a major part of the spa experience. Many people feel they need to leave their home and the cares of the day behind. While it is important to create an ambience that feels different from your daily routine, with a little planning, a few props, and some clearly expressed boundaries with your family, you will be able to transform your home into a wonderful environment for relaxation. This can be accomplished quite easily and inexpensively, too.

Separate the Making from the Enjoying

It is so important to set things up in such a way that you get the full value of the experience while still doing it yourself. Whenever possible, separate the process of creating the products from the time set aside to use them. I really enjoy creating herbal products; the alchemist in me enjoys experimenting. Yet when it's time to use the products, out comes the inner princess. So by all means, enjoy the creation process and allow yourself to become fully absorbed in making your treatments. But remember also to allow yourself to switch gears, to let go of the "creator" role for a while, and luxuriate in the spa treatments when the time is right.

A SPECIAL MESSAGE FOR WOMEN

Women are drawn to spas because they provide one of their few opportunities to receive divinely feminine care. Too many women feel depleted because they themselves don't take the time to receive, because they are caught up in giving to others. This is especially true of mothers. If this rings true for you, accept this as a personal invitation to take in and receive the pleasures of nature.

If you find yourself resenting the people in your life, it may be because you never learned, first, how to give to yourself and, second, how to receive from them. Start taking more time for yourself and I promise that you will see a major change for the better in your relationships and even in your "luck." The busiest of women can and should find 5 to 10 minutes each day for personal pampering.

Open Yourself to the Experience

Part of the spa experience is being able to let go and take in the gifts that the herbs, flowers, and other ingredients have to offer you. My experience with plants is that their healing qualities and individuality are best expressed when you are open to receiving them. Being open to taking in the physical touch of a massage, rub, soak, or other treatment is also key to appreciating the spa experience.

Create the Mood

The key ingredients to create a setting that is relaxing are: lighting, music, color, aroma, comfortable surroundings and privacy, as well as gentle touch.

Lighting. Soft lighting sets a relaxing tone and is helpful in creating ambience. If you need brighter light to actually see what you're doing during the treatment, use a lamp or small light for the immediate area, and dim background lighting. Draping harsh lamps with a scarf can dim the light and set the mood for relaxation.

Candles are another great mood setter. Use care in placing the candles to avoid starting a fire. Candles are also a great way to diffuse fragrances you find calming. Aromatherapy candles abound, or you can simply add a few drops of your favorite scent to a candle. I like to use hurricane candles; they seem safer to me.

Music. Soft, relaxing music helps to set the mood. Some people prefer the peace of silence; for others, classical music is what really settles them down. I love silence, but that's not always possible to achieve, especially if you're doing the treatments when others are at home or if you live in a city or a noisy neighborhood. It is best to avoid music with lyrics, because singing along becomes an outward expression and we want to create the opposite. It pays to invest in a compact disc or two of music you find relaxing; try some of the New Age recordings. The music of Rob Whitesides-Woo or Kitaro takes me to a dreamy place. I also find most flute music soothing. Try several different selections to see what you find most relaxing.

Color. The color of your surroundings will also affect your mood. Recently, a local prison decided to paint the walls pink because this color discourages aggression and seems to foster relaxation. Color is used extensively in the fast-food and formal restaurant businesses: Reds, oranges, and golds stimulate appetite. Pink promotes relaxation. Chose a pink that is pleasing to you: Icy, hot, rosy, pastel, peach, coral, and salmon will all work. Hate pink? Choose a soft color that you love.

Drape the color around the area where you will be pampered. Throw a pink scarf over the lampshade and dim the light while bringing in the color at the same time. Or be really bold and decorate the room that you will be using for treatments in colors you find relaxing. The bathroom is a great place to create a sanctuary.

Aroma. Scents and aromas affect your mood. With the wide availability of pure essential oils and other aromatherapy products, you can easily create a scent atmosphere at home. Choose a fragrance that you find pleasing and calming. A scent may have a different effect on different people, depending on associations and life experiences, but lavender and chamomile are the fragrances most often chosen for relaxation. Bergamot, frankincense, neroli, patchouli, rose, sandalwood, and ylang-ylang are also relaxing. Patchouli, sandalwood, and frankincense are earthy; the others are more flowery. Visit a store that carries essential oils and use the tester to sample various scents. *Note:* Essential oils are highly concentrated; most should not be applied directly to the skin.

Comfortable surroundings. You know what this means for you: Maybe you like the casualness of country decor, or a more refined elegance, a dramatic setting, or funky, or art deco. Whatever your preference, create a setting that is both pleasing and offers privacy.

MAKE YOUR SPA EXPERIENCE ENJOYABLE

Pamper yourself! Use

◆ Large, fluffy towels
◆ Tub pillow
◆ Tub tray
◆ Shower stool
◆ Terry cloth robe
◆ Turban
◆ Slippers
◆ Space heater

or anything else that makes your spa special.

CHAPTER 15
Herbs for the Hair and Scalp

Achieving great-looking hair is not difficult, nor does it need to be expensive. With a few common kitchen ingredients and some specialty oils, herbs, and flowers, you can create a variety of treatments that your hair will respond to quickly. The time you invest in creating these easy formulas will be rewarded with healthier, more radiant hair.

You can customize the basic herbal shampoo provided in this chapter to address your particular hair color, texture, and other individual needs. The herbal hair conditioner and rinse formulas should be applied after the shampoo to help keep the hair healthy from the roots to the ends. The scalp treatments here, including a flower essence massage, are designed to keep the scalp and new hair growth healthy. The final section of this chapter offers instructions for herbal hair coloring, a fun area to explore.

SHAMPOOING TECHNIQUE

For best results, try the following:

♦ Wet hair thoroughly and use a small amount of shampoo, a dollop about the size of a quarter.

♦ Put the shampoo on your hands. Rub them together to form a lather before applying to your hair.

♦ Use your fingertips, not your fingernails, to massage the shampoo into your scalp.

♦ Rinse hair thoroughly, then shampoo again.

♦ Rinse again thoroughly, using the coolest water possible for the shiniest hair.

♦ Pat hair dry; avoid rubbing.

♦ Gently comb hair, using a broad-tooth comb.

HERBAL SHAMPOOS

Shampoos are made to clean the scalp first and the hair second. I recommend customizing your shampoo recipe so that it offers optimal nourishment to your particular hair type and condition.

Selecting Customized Herbs for the Basic Shampoo Formula

Choose herbs for your shampoo that will enhance your hair color and texture, and that address any special needs you may have. You can mix and match herbs from the following lists to develop an individualized combination that is best for your hair.

INGREDIENTS FOR DIFFERENT HAIR TYPES

Dry	Normal	Oily	Ethnic
Comfrey root	Dandelion	Watercress	Comfrey
Avocado	Horse tail	Strawberry leaf	Nettle
Elder flowers	Clover	White willow bark	Cherry bark
Orange blossoms		Lemon grass	Olive oil

INGREDIENTS FOR SPECIAL CONDITIONS

Shine	Manage-ability	Softness	Dandruff	Growth
Egg	Yogurt	Cherry bark	White willow bark	St.-John's-wort
Raspberry	Cherry bark	Burdock root	Birch bark	Nettle
Nettle	Beer	Olive oil	Comfrey	Sage
Vinegar		Marjoram	Nettle	Basil
Quassia			Peppermint	Rosemary
			Vinegar	Onion juice

Blond	Brunette	Red	Darkest
Chamomile	Sage	Henna	Black malva
Calendula	Lavender	Calendula	Indigo
Lemon peel	Cinnamon chips	Red hibiscus	Lavender
Honey	Cloves	Cinnamon	Sage
Lemon juice	Rosemary	Beets	
Mullein flowers			

BASIC SHAMPOO FORMULA

¼ cup (60 ml) fresh herbs (2 table-spoons [30 ml] dried)

1 cup (250 ml) spring water

2 tablespoons (30 ml) liquid castile soap

1 teaspoon (5 ml) almond or apricot kernel oil

2 drops essential oil

Yield: Approximately 24 shampoos

To make:

1. Place herbs in a clean 10-ounce (284 g) glass jar with a lid.

2. Boil the spring water and pour over the herbs.

3. Cover and let steep for 10 to 20 minutes.

4. Strain the liquid from the herbs into a bowl.

5. Add the liquid castile soap and almond and mix thoroughly.

6. Scent with essential oil and mix again.

7. Bottle in a plastic container with a spout or a clean recycled shampoo bottle.

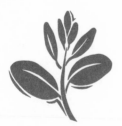

HERBAL HAIR CONDITIONERS

Herbal hair conditioners help make hair more manageable and often impart a smoother and softer texture. They are especially good for those who cannot live without hot rollers, curling irons, and blow dryers.

JOJOBA CONDITIONER

1 cup (250 ml) rose floral water (see recipe on page 254)
1 tablespoon (15 ml) jojoba oil
10 drops vitamin E oil

Yield: 1 treatment for long hair (cut recipe in half for short hair)

To make:
1. In the top of a double boiler, gently warm the rose water.
2. Once rose water is warm, add jojoba oil.
3. Pour the mixture in a blender and add the vitamin E. Blend at high speed for 2 minutes.

To use:
1. Wet hair with warm water.
2. Pour the conditioner onto your hair and scalp, massaging in thoroughly.
3. For damaged hair or extra conditioning, leave on for several minutes, perhaps while bathing.
4. Rinse thoroughly with warm water.
5. Shampoo lightly and rinse again with cool water.

MAYONNAISE HAIR PACK

A longtime favorite of my husband's grandmother Bessie, mayonnaise is a great conditioner for dry hair.

1 cup (250 ml) mayonnaise (make your own fresh or use a premade natural product)

Yield: 1 treatment

To use:

1. Wet hair with warm water.

2. Scoop mayonnaise into a small dish.

3. Dip your fingertips (not nails) into the bowl.

4. Gently massage the mayonnaise all over your scalp, working in a circular motion.

5. Massage the mayonnaise into the hair shaft and the ends.

6. Cover your hair with a plastic bag and allow the mayonnaise to stay on the scalp for at least 30 minutes.

7. Shampoo as you normally would.

8. Repeat weekly, or as often as desired.

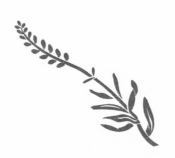

FLOURING

More the rage in Europe, especially France, than in North America, flouring is used for making the hair manageable and shiny. Most any flour will work, but I prefer white spelt and barley for added softness.

½ cup (125 ml) white spelt flour

½ cup (125 ml) barley flour

½ cup (125 ml) distilled water

½ cup (125 ml) rose or lavender floral water (see recipe on page 254)

1 tablespoon (15 ml) apple cider vinegar

1 plastic bag that can fit over the hair

Yield: 1 treatment for long hair

To make:

1. Sift the flours together in a large bowl.

2. Pour the distilled water, floral water, and vinegar over the flours.

To use:

1. Spoon the flour mixture onto dry hair.

2. Smooth the paste all over the hair shaft. (This treatment is for the hair. It is not harmful for the scalp, but the focus is on getting the paste on the individual strands of hair.)

3. Sweep the coated hair up on top of your head and cover with a plastic bag, securing with a hair clip or clothespin.

4. Leave on for 20 to 30 minutes.

5. Remove plastic bag and rinse the mixture off hair thoroughly using cool water. (Hot water will make the flour stick to the hair shafts.)

6. Shampoo as usual; rinse with cool water.

HERBAL HAIR RINSES

Hair rinses are helpful in correcting hair's pH, removing residue from shampoo and other hair products, and creating a healthy-looking shine. Rinses can also bring out the highlights in your hair.

SHINY HAIR RINSE

Using apple cider vinegar and lemon juice is the best treatment for maintaining the natural pH balance of your hair and making it shiny. Omit the lemon juice and double the vinegar if you don't want even the slightest lightening of color.

1 cup (250 ml) water
Juice from ½ lemon
2 tablespoons
(30 ml) apple
cider vinegar

Yield: 1 treatment

To make:
1. Combine all ingredients in a pitcher or jar and mix well.
To use:
1. Shampoo and rinse hair as usual.
2. Pour the mixture on your hair and massage into the scalp and through the hair.
3. Rinse thoroughly with cool water.

BOUNCY HAIR RINSE

This one is so easy to make that anyone can do it — and there's no mixing involved. It's so effective that pretty soon everyone will be calling you Tigger — after Winnie-the-Pooh's bouncy friend!

1 cup (250 ml) beer

Yield: 1 treatment

To make:
1. Pour the beer into a glass and allow it to go flat and get warm.
To use:
1. Shampoo and rinse hair as usual.
2. Pour the flat warm beer on your hair and work it through.
3. Rinse thoroughly with cool water.

DEODORIZING HAIR RINSE

Anyone who has had to clean an animal that has tangoed with a skunk knows this deodorizing trick. Let's hope the odors you'll be trying to remove won't be as strong as skunk! This is great for getting the smell of smoke from your hair.

1 cup (250 ml) tomato juice
2 teaspoons (10 ml) water

Yield: 1 treatment

To make:
1. Combine the tomato juice and water thoroughly in a jar or pitcher.
To use:
1. Shampoo and rinse hair as usual.
2. Pour the tomato juice mixture on your hair and work it through.
3. Rinse thoroughly with cool water.

DANDRUFF RINSE

Restoring the hair to its mildly acid pH can help to clear up dandruff. See a physician if you don't start to see results in 1 to 2 weeks.

1 cup (250 ml) apple cider vinegar
1 cup (250 ml) water
2 tablespoons (30 ml) fresh lemongrass
2 tablespoons (30 ml) fresh nettle
2 tablespoons (30 ml) fresh peppermint

Yield: 7 treatments (1 week)

To make:
1. In a saucepan, bring the apple cider vinegar and water to a boil.
2. Place the herbs in a widemouthed jar.
3. Pour the boiling vinegar and water over the herbs.
4. Cover and steep for 1 week, shaking daily.
5. Strain out the herbs and decant the liquid.
To use:
1. Dilute ¼ cup (60 ml) herbal vinegar mixture with 1 cup (250 mi) water.
2. After shampooing and rinsing hair thoroughly, rinse with diluted vinegar.
3. Let the vinegar sit on the scalp for 1 minute.
4. Rinse thoroughly with cool water.
5. Pat hair dry.

OILY HAIR RINSE

Get out your field guide to gather the material for this one. Wild watercress is delicious to eat and full of vitamins and minerals that are good for the hair. This slightly acid rinse removes residue on the hair, leaving it squeaky clean. Found growing near or in stream and creek beds, watercress is abundant in the Northeast and elsewhere in the United States. You can also purchase it in most grocery stores.

⅔ cup (160 ml) water
1 teaspoon (5 ml) apple cider vinegar
2 cups (500 ml) fresh watercress (wild or cultivated)

Yield: 1 treatment

To make:
1. In a saucepan, warm the water and vinegar.
2. Rinse the watercress, removing any dirt and frayed leaves.
3. Place the watercress in a blender, then pour the warm vinegar water over the herbs.
4. Blend on high speed for 2 minutes.
5. Strain, reserving the liquid.

To use:
1. Use this rinse freshly made, while still warm; the heat helps it work.
2. Shampoo your hair, then rinse well.
3. While hair is still damp, pour the warm mixture onto the hair and scalp.
4. Leave on for 10 minutes.
5. Rinse with cool water.

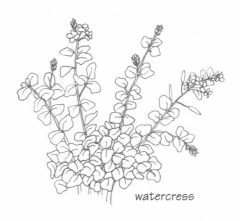

watercress

HERBAL SCALP TREATMENTS

Scalp treatments can rescue damaged hair and solve scalp problems such as dandruff and itchy scalp. Even if you do not have scalp problems, performing an herbal scalp treatment on a monthly basis can result in healthier, more manageable hair and a really clean, invigorated scalp.

OLIVE OIL TREATMENT

Olive oil conditions and improves the strength and elasticity of your hair, so it is a good addition to your shampoo. As a conditioning scalp treatment, the olive oil nourishes new hair. You may substitute other essential oils as you wish.

½ cup (125 ml) olive oil
5 drops frankincense essential oil
5 drops blue chamomile essential oil (optional)
1 plastic bag that can fit over your hair

Yield: 1 or 2 treatments, depending on hair length and thickness

To make:

1. Pour olive oil into a lotion jar, then add the essential oil.

2. Put on lid and shake well to disperse the essential oil.

3. Let sit for 24 hours in a cool, dark place. Shake again before use.

To use:

1. Rinse hair with warm water.

2. Warm 1 tablespoon (15 ml) of the oil in the palms of your hands.

3. Using your fingertips (not nails), gently massage the oil into the scalp in a circular motion.

4. Repeat until the entire scalp has been massaged.

5. Rub the ends of your hair with the remaining oil.

6. Place a plastic bag over your hair, secure by tying or with a hair clip or clothespin, and allow the oil to remain for at least 30 minutes.

7. Rinse well, then shampoo as usual.

HERBAL STEAM

*S*imilar to a facial steam, this treatment encourages circulation around the scalp and promotes healthy hair growth. Steam baths are beneficial for the whole body, but if you don't have one of them, this treatment is a great substitute. If your scalp starts to itch a little, don't worry; this is normal. Your skin is reacting to the increased circulation. When you do a scalp steam weekly, you'll find that the itching sensation gradually fades.

2 quarts (2 liters) water

2 teaspoons (10 ml) dried basil

2 teaspoons (10 ml) dried rose petals

2 teaspoons (10 ml) dried lavender petals

2 teaspoons (10 ml) dried lemon balm

2 teaspoons (10 ml) dried comfrey

Yield: 1 treatment

To make:

1. Bring water to a boil in a large stainless-steel or enamel spaghetti-type pot.

2. Add the dried herbs to the boiling water, cover, and turn off the heat.

3. After 2 minutes, uncover, give the herbs a stir, and remove from the stove.

To use:

1. Place the steaming pot on the floor at the end of your sofa or bed, positioning it so you can lie comfortably with your head 6 to 10 inches above the pot.

2. Loosely pin up your hair, allowing the steam to get to the scalp.

3. Drape a large towel around your hairline and let it hang down around the pot so that it catches the vapors and steam.

4. Keeping your head a comfortable distance from the pot, stay under the towel as long as you comfortably can.

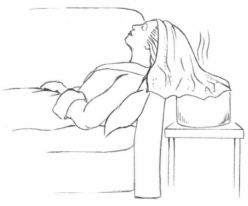

FLOWER ESSENCE SCALP MASSAGE

Flower essences can work wonders to calm the nerves and soothe anyone who is stressed out. The essences are subtle healing substances extracted from flowers. Edward Bach developed a procedure for extracting the essences in the early 1900s. Rescue Remedy, the most popular, is actually a combination of five flower essences and is available in most health food stores. Incorporating flower essences into a scalp treatment benefits both the hair and the emotional and mental state of the recipient. This treatment, which is offered at finer spas, is remarkably easy to make and enjoy at home.

½ cup (125 ml) apricot kernel oil

3 drops red clover flower essence

3 drops lavender flower essence

or

3 drops Rescue Remedy flower essence (or other flower essence combination of your choice)

3 drops lavender essential oil

1 plastic bag that will fit over your hair

Yield: 1 treatment

To make:

1. First add the apricot kernel oil, then the flower essences and essential oils, to a lotion jar.

2. Shake well to disperse all ingredients.

3. Let sit for 24 hours in a cool, dark place; shake again before use.

To use:

1. Rinse hair with warm water.

2. Warm 1 tablespoon (15 ml) of the oil in the palms of your hands.

3. Using your fingertips (not nails), in a circular motion gently massage the oil into the scalp.

4. Repeat until the entire scalp has been massaged.

5. Rub the shafts and ends of your hair with the remaining oil.

6. Place a plastic bag over your hair, secure with a hair clip or clothespin, and allow the oil to remain for at least 30 minutes.

7. Rinse well, then shampoo as you normally would.

DANDRUFF OIL TREATMENT

In treating dandruff, it is important to use an oil treatment for the scalp once each week. The olive oil treatment (see page 223) may be helpful, or try the following. The apple cider vinegar helps to balance the pH of your scalp and the cornmeal gently exfoliates the dry, flaky skin.

½ cup (125 ml) grape-
  seed oil
2 tablespoons (30
  ml) cornmeal
1 tablespoon (15 ml)
  apple cider vinegar
1 plastic bag that will
  fit over your hair

Yield: 1 or 2 treatments,
depending on hair length
and thickness

To make:
1. Pour the grapeseed oil into a bowl, then add the cornmeal and vinegar.
2. Stir well to make a pasty oil.
To use:
1. Rinse hair with warm water.
2. Warm a tablespoon of the oil mixture in the palms of your hands.
3. Using your fingertips (not nails), in a circular motion gently massage the mixture into the scalp.
4. Repeat until the entire scalp has been massaged.
5. Place a plastic bag over your hair, secure with a hair clip or clothespin, and allow the oil to remain for at least 30 minutes.
6. Rinse well, then shampoo as you normally would.

ST.-JOHN'S-WORT AND BASIL OIL SCALP MASSAGE

St.-John's-wort is often used on burns, since it has properties that help regenerate damaged nerves. It is also recommended for stimulating new hair growth for people whose hair has been affected by radiation treatments, pulling, or other damage to the scalp. Basil also encourages hair growth.

Make this oil in midsummer, when the plants are in bloom; it is the flowers that hold the healing powers. The yellow flower and the leaves will turn the oil red. You may also purchase ready-made oil at a health food store.

2 cups (500 ml) fresh St.-John's-wort herb

1 cup (250 ml) fresh basil

3 cups (750 ml) olive oil

10 drops vitamin E oil

5 drops basil essential oil

Yield: 12 applications

To make:

1. Gather the St.-John's-wort in midmorning, when the top of the plant is flowering. Gather the basil before it flowers.

2. Spread the herbs on paper towels and allow to wilt overnight.

3. Stuff the wilted herbs into a large glass jar, packing it as full as possible.

4. Pour the olive oil over the herbs, filling the jar to within ½" of the top.

5. Use a chopstick to poke the herbs and release any captured air or gases.

6. Top off with oil as necessary and screw on the lid of the jar.

7. Store the oil in a dark, cool spot.

8. Repeat steps 5, 6, and 7 daily for 6 days.

9. Let sit for another 6 days; on the 7th day, again repeat steps 5, 6, and 7.

10. Again, let sit for the next 6 days, then on the 7th day repeat steps 5, 6, and 7 again.

11. Let sit for the following 6 days, then strain the herbal material out of the oil and discard it, preserving your oil.

12. Add the vitamin E and basil essential oil to the St.-John's-wort and basil oil mixture, then store in an amber bottle.

To use:

1. Pour 2 tablespoons (30 ml) into a small dish.

2. Dip your fingertips (not nails) into bowl.

3. Gently massage the oil all over your scalp, working in a circular motion.

4. Let the oil stay on the scalp for at least 30 minutes, then shampoo as you normally would.

5. Repeat a few times a week or even every day, if desired.

NATURAL HERBAL HAIR COLORING

Unlike many commercial hair coloring products that damage hair, herbal hair coloring products often condition the hair. So much so, in fact, many people choose to use neutral hennas for their conditioning properties.

FOR BLOND HAIR: LIGHTENING FORMULA

This formula is very effective when applied to light hair shades, but the darker your hair, the harder it will be to lighten it naturally. Persistence is the key. Use this treatment for several sunny days in a row and you're sure to see results.

⅓ cup (80 ml) water
3 tablespoons (45 ml)
　　fresh chamomile flowers
3 tablespoons (45 ml)
　　fresh calendula flowers
Juice from 3 lemons
Broad-brimmed straw hat
　　(an old or inexpensive
　　one that can be cut)
Long white cotton scarf or
　　foot-wide strip of a
　　bedsheet

Yield: 1–2 treatments

To make:
1. Bring the water to a boil.
2. Pour the boiling water over the fresh herbs and let steep for 20 minutes.
3. Strain the infusion, reserving the liquid.
4. Add the lemon juice and mix well.
5. Decant into a spray bottle.
To use:
1. For best results, pick a sunny day to do this treatment.
2. Cut out the top of your broad-brimmed hat. *Note:* If you have short hair, you will not need to use a hat.

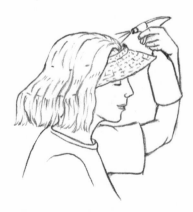

3. Put on the hat. Pull all your hair through the top, letting it spill down over the brim. If necessary, secure the hat using the scarf or bedsheet around the brim. The scarf can also help keep the lemon mixture from dripping down your face.

4. Spray the lemon mixture to thoroughly dampen all your hair.

5. Sit out in the sunshine (be sure to apply protection to other areas of your body). The longer you sit in the sun, the more lightening will occur; try at least 30 minutes and up to 4 hours.

6. As your hair dries, repeat the lemon spray often.

7. Be sure to use a good conditioner — the olive oil or jojoba, for example — after using this treatment, as it tends to be drying.

BLOND HIGHLIGHTING RINSE

The effects of this rinse are subtle. The more you use it, the better the results.

Juice of 1 lemon
¼ cup (60 ml) water

Yield: 1 treatment

To make:

1. Place the lemon juice and water in a glass jar.

2. Shake well.

To use:

1. Shampoo and rinse your hair as usual.

2. Pour the lemon mixture into your hair.

3. Let sit for 5 minutes.

4. Rinse with cool water.

RED HIGHLIGHTING RINSE

1 cup (250 ml) water
1 tablespoon (15 ml)
  alkanet root

Yield: 1 treatment

To make:
1. Bring the water to a boil.
2. Place the alkanet root in a glass jar.
3. Pour boiling water over the alkanet root.
4. Cover and steep for 10 minutes.
5. Strain root from infusion.

To use:
1. Shampoo and rinse hair as usual.
2. Pour the alkanet infusion into your hair, catching the liquid in a basin. Repour the infusion through the hair 10 times.
3. Let your hair sit for 5 minutes.
4. Rinse with cool water.

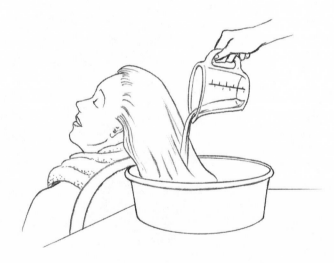

DARKENING HAIR RINSE

1 cup (250 ml) black
   walnut hulls
10 grape leaves
1 cup (250 ml) wine
1 cup (250 ml) water
Cast-iron Dutch oven

Yield: 1 treatment

To make:

1. Place the walnut hulls and grape leaves into the cast-iron Dutch oven.

2. Pour the wine and water over the herbs.

3. Simmer over low heat for 1 hour.

4. Strain, reserving the liquid.

To use:

1. Shampoo and rinse hair as usual.

2. Pour the herbal decoction into your hair, catching the liquid in a basin. Repour the infusion through your hair 10 times.

3. Wait 5 minutes.

4. Rinse with cool water.

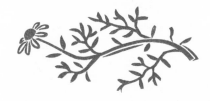

FOR REDHEADS: SHADES OF RED

¼ cup (60 ml) dried calendula flowers
½ cup (125 ml) red henna
⅓ cup (80 ml) boiling water
Rubber gloves
Plastic bag large enough to fit over hair and scalp

Yield: 1 treatment

To make:
1. In a spice mill, powder the calendula petals.
2. Sift together the henna and powdered calendula into a glass or porcelain bowl. (Do not use metal bowls or spoons with henna; the metal will affect the color.)
3. Pour the boiling water over the henna.
4. Mix thoroughly to form a thick paste.

To use:
1. Shampoo and rinse your hair as usual.
2. Wearing rubber gloves, use a wooden or plastic spoon to apply the henna to your hair. Try to avoid getting the henna mixture on your scalp.
3. Still wearing rubber gloves, once the entire head of hair is covered with the henna mixture, massage the henna into your hair to the ends.
4. Wrap the hair on top of your head and cover the hair with the plastic bag, securing it with a hair clip or clothespin.
5. Immediately, using soap, wash off any henna that may have dripped down your face or gotten on your hands or clothing.
6. Let the henna set for 20 to 40 minutes.
7. Rinse your hair thoroughly with warm water until the water runs clear.
8. Shampoo as usual, rinsing well with cool water.

NOTE ON APPLYING HENNA

When applying henna, avoid getting the coloring on your scalp. It will stain the scalp quite heavily. It is inevitable that some henna will get on your scalp, but the less of it, the better. Henna on the scalp will eventually wash out with shampooing, but it's best to minimize the problem by not rubbing any henna mixture into the scalp.

FOR BRUNETTE HAIR: SHADES OF BROWN

There are many henna color choices available these days. Shop around until you find a store with a good selection. You can use just one henna color for this treatment, or mix several shades. Henna will make your hair redder or browner, but not lighter.

2 tablespoons (30 ml) powdered cloves
2 tablespoons (30 ml) quassia bark
½ cup (125 ml) brown henna
⅓ cup (80 ml) boiling water
Rubber gloves
Plastic bag large enough to fit over hair and scalp

Yield: 1 treatment

To make:

1. In a spice mill, powder the cloves and quassia bark.

2. Sift the henna, powdered cloves, and quassia bark together into a glass or porcelain bowl. (Do not use metal bowls or spoons with henna; metal affects the color.)

3. Pour the boiling water over the henna.

4. Mix thoroughly to form a thick paste.

To use:

1. Shampoo and rinse your hair as usual.

2. Wearing rubber gloves, use a wooden or plastic spoon to apply the henna to your hair. Try to avoid getting too much of the mixture on your scalp.

3. Once the entire head of hair is covered with the henna mixture, and still wearing rubber gloves, massage the henna into the hair all the way to the ends.

4. Wrap the hair on top of your head and cover the hair with the plastic bag, securing with a hair clip or clothespin.

5. Immediately, with soap, wash off any henna that may have dripped down your face or gotten on your hands or clothing.

6. Let the henna set on your hair for 20 to 40 minutes.

7. Rinse your hair thoroughly with warm water until the water runs clear.

8. Shampoo as usual, rinsing well with cool water.

CHAPTER 16

Herbal Rituals for a Beautiful Face and Neck

If the eyes are the windows of the soul, then the face is the reflection of the physical being. Facial treatments and skin care have a great impact on your overall appearance and the health of your skin. In this chapter, you'll learn about creating your own facial rituals at home. You may also be surprised to find a plethora of ingredients for facial scrubs and masks in your kitchen right now, without even going to the grocery store.

Once you begin making the recipes in this chapter, the only lotions or skin creams you'll need to buy will be for sunscreen purposes, although you can try your hand at making those yourself, as well. The ritual of creating floral waters may become an enjoyable part of your life, as may the process of creating astringents, face washes, and even aftershaves for all members of your family.

HERBAL EYE TREATMENTS

The eyes are the most delicate area on your face. They are also its focal point, and it's important to treat your eyes tenderly. Eye packs are easy applications to combine with other treatments such as a foot massage and a body wrap.

APPLYING EYE TREATMENT

In applying creams, lotions, and eye makeup, it's worth taking a bit of extra care so that you keep the skin around your eyes looking as healthy as possible. Following are the application steps I suggest:

1. Dab the product of choice onto your ring finger.
2. Gently pat the lotion, under the eye, starting at the outside and working in.
3. Next pat the lotion on top of the eye, again starting at the outside and working in.

Note: Working in the other direction, from inside to outside, encourages crow's-feet wrinkles.

VIOLET EYE CREAM

～～～～～

Tired of spending a fortune on eye creams? This recipe is great for tired, puffy, or irritated eyes — or just for day-to-day makeup removal. This exquisite formula is very popular; as a matter of fact, I just made 24 jars of cream for my dear friend Maria. The blue chamomile essential oil is expensive (approximately $50 for ½ ounce). It's high in azulene — an anti-inflammatory agent extracted from chamomile flowers — and it's very soothing to the delicate area around the eye. It's not crucial for the recipe, but a great addition when you can afford the indulgence. If you are allergic to chamomile tea, leave it out.

½ cup (125 ml) fresh violet flowers

½ cup (125 ml) fresh violet leaves

1¼ cups (310 ml) almond oil

½ cup (125 ml) fresh horsetail

2 tablespoons (30 ml) beeswax

10 drops vitamin E oil

10 drops blue chamomile essential oil (optional)

Yield: Approximately 30 ¼-ounce containers

To make:

1. Gather the violet flowers and leaves and place them on a towel to wilt overnight.

2. In a double boiler, steep the leaves, petals, and horsetail in oil over low heat for 5 hours.

3. Grate the beeswax or cut into small pieces.

4. Strain the plant material from the oil completely.

5. Pour the oil back into the double boiler, adding the grated beeswax.

6. Melt the beeswax into the oil completely, then remove from heat.

7. Quickly add the vitamin E and blue chamomile oil.

8. Pour into dainty ¼-ounce (7 g) containers or jars.

9. Decorate with violet stickers.

To use, refer to Applying Eye Treatment box.

～～～～～

BE SELECTIVE ABOUT YOUR UTENSILS

In all your herbal preparations, the type of cooking utensils you use is important. Use nonreactive utensils made of stainless steel, glass, or enamel. Do not use aluminum, copper, or cast iron; these metals will affect the finished product.

▲▲▲▲▲

CUCUMBER EYE PACK

Cucumbers have long been known to sooth puffy eyes. We've all seen in magazines the models with cucumbers on their eyes, so what's the hesitation? It doesn't get much easier than this!

¼ cucumber

Yield: 1 treatment

To make:
1. Slice the cucumber to fit over eyes.
2. If you really like things simple, cut just two slices. I prefer to slice 5 to 10 extremely thin slices and use several on each eye. Either method works.

To use:
1. Spritz eye area with water.
2. Lying down, place cucumber slices on your eyelids and leave in place for 5–10 minutes.

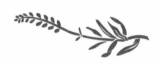

BAGGY EYE TREATMENT

Raw potato slices will help tighten baggy, puffy eyes. All you need is a potato and a knife or slicer!

¼ potato

Yield: 1 treatment

To make:
1. Slice the potato to fit over your eyes.
2. Cut 2 slices, or, if you prefer, 5 to 10 very thin slices, several for each eye. Either method works.

To use:
1. Spritz eye area with water.
2. Lying down, place the potato slices on your eyelids and leave in place for at least 10 minutes for best results.

CROW'S-FEET TREATMENT

Here's another treatment that's easy to whip up! Egg whites help plump and firm wrinkled skin.

1 egg white
Cotton ball

Yield: 1 treatment

To make:
1. Beat the egg white to just before it forms soft peaks.

To use:
1. Dab the egg white in a crescent shape around the eye, along the cheekbone and the outer eye area.
2. Allow to sit for 10 minutes.
3. Spritz the egg white with water.
4. Using cool water on a cotton ball, gently remove.

HERBAL EYELASH AND BROW TREATMENTS

The eyelashes and brows, like any hairs on your body, respond to the moisturizing effects of natural oils. Pampering these eye hairs makes them healthier and more manageable, and bolder looking without the need for mascara or brow pencil.

NOURISHING OIL

Castor bean oil is nourishing for the eyelashes and brows. If you are sensitive to mascara, as I am, this recipe is a good substitute for accentuating the natural color of your lashes. You can use this application daily, and once applied, it can be left on all day.

Cotton swab
1 teaspoon (5 ml) castor bean oil

Yield: 1 treatment

To use:
1. Dab the cotton swab into the oil and apply to the lashes only, being careful not to get any oil on the skin surrounding the eye.
2. Dab the eyebrow where it is most thickly haired.
3. Using your ring finger, gently rub the oil over the entire eyebrow.

HERBAL EYE PILLOW

⌄⌄⌄

This little eye pillow blocks light and provides slight weight and pressure, which will relax the eyes and facial muscles, thus reducing tension, stimulating circulation, and relieving mild headaches. If you have a sewing machine and can stitch a straight seam, you can easily make your own version that matches any store-bought ones. You can wash the cover without having to clean the entire pillow.

¼ yard (23 cm) silky, natural, washable fabric (silk or cotton is best)

1 cup (250 ml) flaxseed

½ cup (125 ml) lavender flowers

3 drops essential oil of lavender (optional)

Yield: One eye pillow

To make:

1. Choose a fabric in a color that is soothing to you.

2. Fold the fabric in half, right sides together, and trace eye pillow and cover patterns onto the wrong side of the fabric. Cut on the lines.

3. With right sides together, stitch a ½" (1¼ cm) seam around the long sides and one end of the pillow. Turn right side out. Stitch the two long sides, and one short end of the cover as well. Hem the edges of the open end by hand or machine.

4. Mix the flaxseed and lavender (adding the scent, if desired).

5. Stuff the pillow with the flower and seed mixture.

6. Hand-sew the remaining side closure.

To use:

1. Squeeze the eye pillow to release the soothing lavender scent.

2. Place the eye pillow in the washable cover.

3. Place over the eyes while relaxing or receiving another treatment.

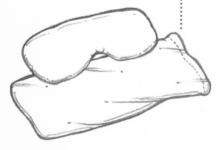

HERBAL LIP TREATMENTS

Do you know someone who seems "addicted" to a commercial lip treatment product? The product may contain chemicals that are irritating to the lips, encouraging continued use of the product. To avoid commercial lip balm addictions, make your own pure, simple products that you will be free to use as needed.

LIP BALM

These are a snap to make, and the recipe lends itself to numerous variations. Use an infused oil to incorporate the healing properties of herbs into your balm (see pages 50–51). Pam Montgomery taught me this basic recipe, which we made green in our apprenticeship class. I prefer to add the alkanet, which yields a range of shades from red to pink to spicy and also adds emollient benefits. It's a great project to do with children; let each one choose a pretty sticker to decorate the dainty container. These make great party favors, too.

LIP BALM RECIPE VARIATIONS

Banana. Omit alkanet root and use banana flavoring oil.
Cinnamon. Use an oil infused with plantain and comfrey and add cinnamon flavoring.
Cherry Red. Double the amount of alkanet root for a deep red color and add cherry flavoring.

Use your imagination and develop your own variations.

½ cup (125 ml) oil (apricot kernel, almond, or grapeseed)
2 tablespoons (30 ml) grated beeswax
½ teaspoon (2½ ml) alkanet root
10 drops natural flavoring oil
3 drops vitamin E oil
Stickers

Yield: Approximately 15 ¼-ounce (7-gram) containers

To make:

1. In a double boiler, gently heat oil to melt the beeswax.
2. Add enough alkanet root for desired redness. (Oil should look black for a deep red color and red for a lighter shade.)
3. When beeswax is entirely melted, strain the oil into an easy-pour measuring cup, removing the alkanet root from the mix.
4. Add the natural flavoring oil and vitamin E and pour into containers.

LIP WRINKLE WONDER

Papaya is great for diminishing wrinkles around the lips.

¼ very ripe papaya **or**
¼ cup (60 ml)
papaya juice

Yield: 1 treatment

To make:
1. Mash the papaya into a mushy pulp.
To use:
1. Lie down with a towel behind your head and your hair pulled back.
2. Generously apply the papaya mush to your lips and the surrounding area. If you are using juice, apply to a cotton ball and dab the area around your lips. (This is also great for breakout-prone areas such as the T-zone.)
3. Leave on for 10 minutes; follow with a facial exfoliation treatment (see pages 268–271).
4. Rinse with cool water.

DAILY CLEANSERS

These gentle products are great for daily use and a fresh, clean feel. The following recipes were inspired by and adapted from Connie Krochmal's *Natural Cosmetics from Beehive to Herb Garden.*

HERBAL CLEANSING MILK FOR DRY SKIN

2 tablespoons (30 ml) dried calendula
2 tablespoons (30 ml) dried chamomile blossoms
2 tablespoons (30 ml) dried comfrey
2 tablespoons (30 ml) dried lemon balm
2 tablespoons (30 ml) dried rose petals
1 tablespoon (15 ml) bee pollen

1 cup (250 ml) boiling water
¼ cup (60 ml) aloe vera gel
½ cup (125 ml) glycerin
2 tablespoons (30 ml) honey
10 drops vitamin E oil

Yield: 4 treatments

To make:
1. Place the dried flowers and herbs and bee pollen in a 10-ounce (284-gram) glass jar with lid.
2. Pour the boiling water over the flowers and pollen, cover, and steep for 20 minutes.

3. Strain out herbs, reserving the liquid.

4. Pour the liquid into a blender and add the remaining ingredients.

5. Blend at high speed for 2 minutes.

6. Pour into a widemouthed jar.

7. Keep refrigerated; mixture will last 1 week.

APPLYING FACIAL CLEANSERS

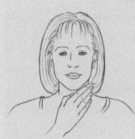
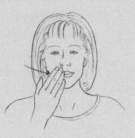
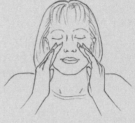

1. Apply cleanser to the throat using gentle strokes across the neck from side to side, starting at the upper shoulders and moving up.

2. Apply to the face with a side-to-side motion, gently swiping across the chin, above the lips, and then across the forehead.

3. Using your fingertips, gently massage in upward strokes. Start at the jaw outside the mouth, coming up along the side of the nose and across the bridge of the nose.

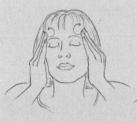
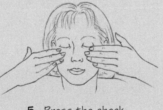
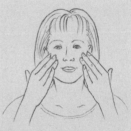

4. Make several spiraling, circular motions spanning the entire forehead, ending up above and outside the eyes.

5. Press the cheekbones with very light pressure, moving from the outer side inward.

6. Use a spiral, circular stroke on the cheeks.

Repeat steps 1 through 6. Using a warm facecloth (or a diaper!), cover your entire face and gently dab all over. Rinse with cool water.

HERBAL CLEANSING MILK FOR NORMAL SKIN

2 tablespoons (30 ml) dried elder flower blossoms

2 tablespoons (30 ml) dried rose petals

2 tablespoons (30 ml) dried lavender

2 tablespoons (30 ml) dried calendula

2 tablespoons (30 ml) dried comfrey

1 tablespoon (15 ml) bee pollen

1 cup (250 ml) boiling water

¼ cup (60 ml) aloe vera gel

¼ cup (60 ml) glycerin

¼ cup (60 ml) honey

10 drops vitamin E oil

Yield: 4 treatments

To make:

1. Place the dried herbs and flowers and bee pollen in a 10-ounce (284-gram) glass jar with lid.

2. Pour the boiling water over the flowers and pollen; cover and steep for 20 minutes.

3. Strain, reserving the liquid.

4. Pour the liquid into a blender and add the remaining ingredients.

5. Blend at high speed for 2 minutes.

6. Pour into a widemouthed jar.

7. Keep refrigerated; mixture will last 1 week.

To use, refer to the Applying Facial Cleansers box.

HERBAL CLEANSING GEL FOR OILY SKIN

2 tablespoons (30 ml) dried parsley

2 tablespoons (30 ml) dried rose petals

2 tablespoons (30 ml) dried rosemary

2 tablespoons (30 ml) dried calendula

2 tablespoons (30 ml) dried linden blossoms

1 cup (250 ml) boiling water

½ cup (125 ml) aloe vera gel

¼ tablespoon (4 ml) honey

10 drops vitamin E oil

Yield: 4 treatments

To make:

1. Place the dried flowers and herbs in a 10-ounce (284-gram) glass jar with lid.

2. Pour the boiling water over the flowers; cover and steep for 20 minutes.

3. Strain, reserving the liquid.

4. Pour the liquid into a blender and add the remaining ingredients.

5. Blend at high speed for 2 minutes.

6. Pour into a widemouthed jar.

7. Keep refrigerated; mixture will last 1 week.

To use, refer to the Applying Facial Cleansers box.

FACIAL STEAMS

How do you think those movie stars stay so beautiful? Well, you say you want movie-star results but you don't have a movie-star budget? Don't fret. You don't need any fancy equipment to hydrate your face — just a large pot of water, a big towel, and a selection of herbs. Receiving a facial in a salon is a wonderful treat, but you don't have to wait for an appointment when you do it at home. These treatments are very easy.

Many students of aesthetics have told me what a difference they noted in their skin after serving as facial steam guinea pigs in classes over the course of a semester. Facial steams are recommended on a weekly basis.

BASIC HERBAL FACIAL STEAM

You may find that your face gets itchy the first time you steam it. This is normal; your skin is reacting to the increased circulation caused by the steam. If you give yourself a facial steam weekly, you'll find that the itching sensation will decrease gradually, and the increased circulation will have your face all aglow.

2 quarts (2 liters) water
1 cup (250 ml) dried
   herbs
Large spaghetti-type pot

Yield: 1 treatment

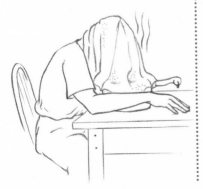

To make:
1. Bring water to a boil in a large pot.
2. Add dried herb mixture to the boiling water, cover, and turn off the heat.
3. After 2 minutes, uncover, give the herbs a stir, and remove from the stove.
To use:
1. Place the pot on a table or counter where you can sit comfortably with your face about 6 inches above it. Drape a large towel over your head and allow it to hang down around the pot so that it catches the vapors and steam.
2. Keeping a comfortable distance from the pot, try to stay under the towel as long as you comfortably can.

HERBAL FACE LIFT

Remember this recipe the next time you're getting ready to go to your high school reunion! It's very effective at tightening the skin under the chin and the neck and can also reduce some of the roundness in your cheeks. This recipe is too drying for the eye area, which has no oil ducts; avoid applying it there. Use Violet Eye Cream (see recipe on page 235) to plump up the skin around the eyes.

½ cup (125 ml) baking soda
½ cup (125 ml) orrisroot
¼ cup (60 ml) sea salt
2 tablespoons (30 ml) dulse
2 tablespoons (30 ml) kelp
½ cup (125 ml) distilled water
Several strips of 8" by 8' (20 cm by 2.4 m) torn bedsheets, gauze, or other clean cotton material

Yield: 1 treatment

To make:

1. Sift together the baking soda, orrisroot, and sea salt into a large bowl.

2. In a spice mill, powder the dulse and kelp and add to the dry ingredients.

3. Heat the distilled water to boiling, then pour over the dry ingredients.

4. Stir thoroughly.

To use:

1. Wear a shirt with a fairly low neckline for easy access to your neck and chin.

2. Moisturize the jaw, chin, neck, and cheek area of your face with a light moisturizer or vegetable oil. Dab your face with a cloth to remove any excess oil or moisturizer.

3. Using a wooden spoon, apply the mixture to the jaw, chin, neck, and cheeks.

FACIAL STEAM HERB SUGGESTIONS

Use any of the herbs listed for your skin type, or a combination.

Dry skin: rose, lavender, comfrey, chamomile

Normal skin: rose, lavender, lemon balm, calendula

Oily skin: rosemary, sage, witch hazel

Problem (dull or breakout-prone) skin: comfrey

4. Immediately wrap the sheets or gauze snuggly first around the neck, then from the chin around the head several times, to just below the eyes. Next, wrap sheet or gauze up over top of head and under the chin a few times to secure. I like to combine this treatment with the cucumber eye treatment. Another option is to soak cotton balls in floral water or a natural oil and to place them on the closed eyelids.

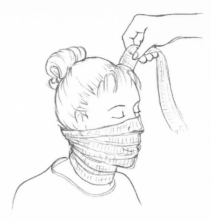

5. Relax and be quiet until the mixture and sheets become dry and tight (approximately 30 minutes). No talking — this will stretch the sheets and keep you from getting the results you desire.

6. Rinse your face and neck with the coldest water you can bear. Notice the surprising softening effects on your skin.

PAPAYA ENZYME TREATMENT

This treatment is used in conjunction with a facial steam to help clear up blemishes.

1 very ripe papaya

Yield: 1 treatment

To make:
1. Mash the papaya into a mushy pulp.
To use:
1. Prepare a facial steam according to the recipe on page 243.
2. Generously apply the papaya mush to your face, being careful to avoid the eyes.
3. Steam your face with the papaya on it following the instructions for the facial steam.

HERBAL SCRUBS AND MASKS

Nuts and grains are popular ingredients in facial scrubs and masks. Aduki beans, oatmeal, barley, garbanzo beans, and even poppy seeds help to exfoliate the skin. Nuts are particularly good if you have dry skin because of their high fat content. Recipes for a few facial scrubs and masks follow, but again, please don't limit yourself to just these ingredients. If there is a commercial product you like, look at the ingredients and try your hand at creating a similar product at home — without the added chemical preservatives.

APPLYING FACIAL PRODUCTS

For best results and to minimize aging effects, apply products to the face by using upward and outward strokes. Apply products with your fingertips (not fingernails) in small, circular motions. Use only your ring finger anywhere near your eyes and use inward strokes. The eye area has the most delicate skin and the ring finger is the weakest finger, thus discouraging crow's-feet.

AVENA FACIAL GRAINS

These grains can be packaged in a pretty glass spice jar with a shaker top. Decorate with stickers and ribbon for a beautiful gift. This recipe was inspired by Rosemary Gladstar's "Miracle Grains." I've used the oat bran and poppy seeds for gentle exfoliation. This recipe may be easily doubled for gift-giving.

½ cup (125 ml) oat-meal

¼ cup (60 ml) oat bran

3 tablespoons (45 ml) almonds

½ cup (125 ml) white clay

2 tablespoons (30 ml) poppy seeds

2 tablespoons (30 ml) dried herbs

Yield: 16 treatments

To make:

1. In a blender or spice/coffee mill, grind the oatmeal and oat bran, leaving some grit.

2. Grind the almonds and strain, leaving a bit of grit for exfoliation of the skin.

3. Combine with all other ingredients in a large bowl, using a wire whisk to mix.

4. Package in four 1-ounce spice jars.

To use:

1. Combine 1 tablespoon (15 ml) grains with 1 tablespoon (15 ml) water, milk, or yogurt and mix into a paste.

2. Apply to face by rubbing gently and in a circular motion. Especially treat the T-zone: This is the often oily area of the face that includes the forehead, nose, mouth, and chin (which form a T shape).

3. Rinse with warm water and then with cooler water.

HERBS FOR FACIAL GRAINS

Dry skin: rose, lavender

Normal skin: rose, lavender, lemon balm, calendula

Oily skin: rosemary, sage, witch hazel

Problem (dull or breakout-prone) skin: Use green clay instead of white and add 1 teaspoon (5 ml) goldenseal, 1 teaspoon (5 ml) myrrh, and 1 teaspoon (5 ml) comfrey root

OXYGEN FACIAL

This treatment is the latest rage at many top spas. The recipe contains hydrogen peroxide, which releases oxygen as it is combined with the other ingredients and applied to the skin. Oxygen helps slow the aging process. Be sure to make it fresh for best results.

⅛ cup (30 ml) oatmeal
1 tablespoon (15 ml) almonds
1 tablespoon (15 ml) white clay
1 teaspoon (5 ml) dried rose petals
1 tablespoon (15 ml) hydrogen peroxide
3 tablespoons (45 ml) water

Yield: 1 treatment

To make:

1. In a blender or spice/coffee mill, grind the oatmeal, leaving some grit.

2. Grind the almonds and strain, leaving a bit of grit for exfoliation of the skin.

3. Combine all dry ingredients in a large bowl, using a wire whisk to mix.

To use:

1. In a small bowl, combine the oatmeal mixture with the hydrogen peroxide and water, and form into a paste.

2. Apply to face by rubbing gently in a circular motion.

3. Allow to set on the face for 5 minutes.

4. Rinse with cool water.

HERBAL TREATMENTS FOR BLACKHEADS

Use this treatment in conjunction with the facial steam to help clear up blackheads.

¼ cup (50 ml) parsley

Yield: 1 treatment

To make:

1. Juice the parsley in a juicer or blender.

To use:

1. Prepare a facial steam according to the instructions on page 243.

2. Generously apply the parsley juice and pulp to the areas on your face that are prone to blackheads, avoiding the eyes.

3. Steam your face with the parsley juice on it, following the instructions for facial steams.

PEEL-OFF MASK

I bet you didn't think you could create one of these fancy masks at home. Good news! Since they contain primarily gelatin, herbal infusion, and juice, peel-off masks are quite simple to make. This recipe was inspired by and adapted from Janice Cox's *Natural Beauty at Home.*

¼ cup (60 ml) fruit juice

¼ cup (60 ml) herbal infusion (see page 292)

1 packet unflavored gelatin

Yield: 1 treatment

To make:

1. Pour the liquid ingredients into an oven-proof glass container.

2. Add the gelatin, stirring to dissolve completely.

3. Gently heat the mixture in a double boiler for 1 minute, stirring constantly.

4. Refrigerate the mixture for 30 minutes.

To use:

1. Spread a thin layer over your face and allow it to dry.

2. Peel off and rinse with cool water.

3. Pat dry.

JUICE AND HERBAL INFUSION SUGGESTIONS FOR PEEL-OFF MASK

Sensitive and fair skin: apple juice with rose petal infusion

Dry skin: honeydew or cantaloupe juice with lemon balm infusion

Normal skin: raspberry juice with raspberry leaf infusion

Oily skin: watermelon juice with rosemary infusion

Breakout-prone skin: tomato juice with garlic infusion

LOTIONS AND POTIONS

Many of us spend a fortune on face and body creams and lotions. The following recipes are exquisite and though they are a bit tricky, they are by far my most-sought-after products. I call them face creams, but they are affordable enough to make and use for your whole body. Although they do go on a little greasy, your skin will be hydrated by the pure vegetable ingredients, unlike many of the mineral oil products currently on the market. These moisturizers were inspired by Rosemary Gladstar's work; I hope you enjoy my modifications to the basic cream.

ROSE PINK FACE MOISTURIZER

This is my best-seller. You may omit the alkanet root if you don't want the pink color, although alkanet does offer some sunscreen protection. Everyone loves this recipe, but it's especially good for dry skin.

⅔ cup (150 ml) grape-
   seed oil
⅓ cup (75 ml) coconut
   oil
1 teaspoon (5 ml)
   cocoa butter
1 tablespoon (15 ml)
   beeswax
½ teaspoon (2½ ml)
   alkanet root
⅓ cup (75 ml) rose
   water
⅓ cup (75 ml) distilled
   water
⅓ cup (75 ml) aloe
   vera gel
20 drops vitamin E oil
8 drops rose essential
   oil or attar of roses
15 1-ounce (25-gram)
   jars
Yield: Fifteen 1-ounce
(25-gram) jars

To make:
1. In a double boiler, melt grapeseed oil, coconut oil, cocoa butter, beeswax, and alkanet root.
2. Once the beeswax is melted, strain out alkanet root and pour oil mixture into a glass measuring cup, preferably one with a spout.
3. Let cool to room temperature for approximately 1 hour.
4. Set up 15 clean jars on the edge of your counter for easy pouring.
5. Combine the rose water, distilled water, aloe vera gel, vitamin E, and essential oil in the blender and turn to the highest speed for a minute or two.
6. In a slow, thin drizzle, pour the cooled oils into the vortex of the waters while the blender is still going.
7. Listen to the blender; when it chokes, the water and oil have combined.
8. Pour into the jars and decorate with stickers and ribbons.

LAVENDER BLUE FACE MOISTURIZER

This cream contains blue chamomile essential oil, which adds a hint of color along with its healing and regenerative properties. Some people don't care for the scent of the blue chamomile, so smell it first. It is also quite expensive. Although it is very good for your skin, I would never recommend you use a scent that you find unpleasant. Frankincense essential oil also contributes regenerative properties.

⅔ cup (150 ml) grape-
   seed oil
⅓ cup (75 ml) coconut
   oil
1 teaspoon (5 ml)
   cocoa butter
1 tablespoon (30 ml)
   beeswax
⅓ cup (75 ml) lavender
   water
⅓ cup (75 ml) distilled
   water
⅓ cup (75 ml) aloe
   vera gel
20 drops vitamin E oil
5 drops blue chamomile
   essential oil
5 drops lavender
   essential oil
5 drops frankincense
   essential oil
15 1-ounce (25-gram)
   jars

Yield: Fifteen 1-ounce
(25-gram) jars

To make:

1. In a double boiler, melt the grapeseed oil, coconut oil, cocoa butter, and beeswax.

2. Once the beeswax is melted, pour the oil mixture into a glass measuring cup, preferably one with a spout.

3. Let cool to room temperature for approximately 1 hour.

4. Set up 15 clean jars on the edge of your counter for easy pouring.

5. Combine the lavender water, distilled water, aloe vera gel, vitamin E, and essential oils in the blender and turn to the highest speed for a minute or two.

6. In a slow, thin drizzle, pour the cooled oils into the vortex of the waters while the blender is still going.

7. Listen to the blender; when it chokes, the water and oil have combined.

8. Pour into the jars and decorate with stickers and ribbons.

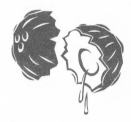

ORANGE BLOSSOM FACE CREAM

Emollient and hydrating, this is a cheery skin cream. The sesame oil in this recipe is a bit greasier than the grapeseed oil used in the other face cream recipes, and it has a stronger scent, but it adds sunscreen protection. Be sure to use cold pressed sesame oil, which will have a lighter scent than the toasted sesame oil found in the international cooking section of your local store.

⅔ cup (160 ml) sesame oil

⅓ cup (80 ml) coconut oil

1 teaspoon (5 ml) cocoa butter

1 tablespoon (15 ml) beeswax

1 teaspoon (5 ml) alkanet root

3 tablespoons (45 ml) calendula

⅓ cup (80 ml) orange blossom water

⅓ cup (80 ml) distilled water

⅓ cup (80 ml) aloe vera gel

20 drops vitamin E oil

10 drops orange blossom essential oil

15 1-ounce (25-gram) jars

Yield: Fifteen 1-ounce (25-gram) jars

To make:

1. In a double boiler, melt the sesame oil, coconut oil, cocoa butter, beeswax, alkanet root, and calendula.

2. Once the beeswax is melted, strain out the alkanet root and pour the oil mixture into a glass measuring cup, preferably one with a spout.

3. Let cool to room temperature for approximately 1 hour.

4. Set up 15 clean jars on the edge of your counter for easy pouring.

5. Combine the orange blossom water, distilled water, aloe vera gel, vitamin E, and essential oil in the blender and turn to the highest speed for a minute or two.

6. In a slow, thin drizzle, pour the cooled oils into the vortex of the water while the blender is still going.

7. Listen to the blender; when it chokes, the water and oil have combined.

8. Pour in the jars and decorate with stickers and ribbons.

FLORAL WATERS

While you can buy aromatic floral waters (also called herbal waters or hydrosols), I find making my own to be an enchanting practice. Floral waters are distilled waters that are all natural and lightly scented. They are wonderful additions to any herbal product, especially moisturizing creams. Less concentrated than essential oils and therefore safe for use undiluted, hydrosols offer many of the same benefits as essential oils. You don't need a lot of sophisticated equipment to make floral waters at home. Once you figure out the arrangement of materials in this homemade "still," it all works almost effortlessly. I like to make floral waters when I plan to be working in the kitchen on something else. While I am preparing meals or other herbal preparations, I can keep an eye on the temperature of the herbal water and the ice and still get other things accomplished.

SUGGESTIONS FOR FLORAL WATERS

Any aromatic herbs will work in this venture. My favorites are rose, lavender, sage, marjoram, lemon balm, any of the mints, and lovage. Be creative!

◆ **For dry skin,** try rose and lavender.
◆ **For normal skin,** try lemon balm and mints.
◆ **For oily skin,** try sage, rosemary, and lovage.

AROMATIC FLORAL WATER

Large pot (12 to 16 quarts)
1 clean brick or flat rock
Bunch of fresh aromatic herbs or flowers (approximately ½ gallon or 2 pounds)
Glass bowl that fits down inside the pot (with 1" clearance around sides)
Water
Stainless-steel bowl large enough to sit on top of the large pot
1 large chunk of ice

Yield: Varies from 2 to 5 oz.

To make:

1. Place the large pot on the stove.

2. Place the brick in the center of the pot.

3. Arrange the fresh herbal material around the brick.

4. Add water up to the top of the brick. This will cover the herbs or flowers.

5. Place the glass bowl on top of the brick. This is where the distilled floral water will collect.

6. Set the stainless-steel bowl on top of the pot and add a large chunk of ice to the bowl. It is best to use one large chunk of ice created by filling a plastic jug with water and then freezing. Smaller ice cubes, while workable, tend to melt faster and require more attention than the big chunk.

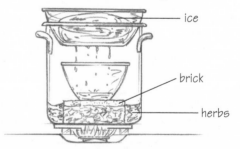

7. Turn the stove burner on low. Gently simmer the herbal mixture on the lowest heat (use a flame tamer if you have a gas range) for approximately 3 hours, taking care that there is always ice in the top. After 3 hours, remove the cover and enjoy the intoxicating aroma wafting through your home. The floral water will have collected in the glass bowl. Bottle this water in a capped container. Use it as a toner (especially good for dry skin) or an astringent, or add it to a face cream recipe.

HERBAL ASTRINGENTS AND AFTERSHAVES

Herbal astringents and aftershaves are used to tone the skin after cleansing. Many astringents contain floral waters and some sort of alcohol, both of which balance the pH of the skin and remove impurities.

QUEEN OF HUNGARY WATER

This recipe was developed for the Queen of Hungary in 1370. It's a wonderful astringent for those with normal, oily, or problem skin, and it's especially good for people with itchy skin. It's touted as the first herbal product to be produced and marketed. Although I include it with astringents, it was used by the Gypsies for almost everything you can think of, from mouthwash to hair rinse to footbaths. I like to use it in the bath. This recipe is best made with fresh herbs.

5 tablespoons (75 ml) fresh lemon balm

4 tablespoons (60 ml) fresh roses

4 tablespoons (60 ml) fresh chamomile

3 tablespoons (45 ml) fresh calendula

3 tablespoons (45 ml) fresh comfrey

1 tablespoon (15 ml) fresh lemon peel

1 tablespoon (15 ml) fresh rosemary

8–10 ounces (227–284 g) apple cider vinegar

Yield: 10 ounces

To make:

1. Place all the fresh herbs in a 12-ounce (340-gram) jar. Completely cover with vinegar.

2. Cover the jar and let sit in a warm spot for 4 weeks, shaking occasionally.

3. Strain the liquid.

4. If desired, combine with floral water of your choice.

QUEEN OF HUNGARY WATER BLENDS

To make a superior astringent, combine Queen of Hungary Water with a floral water that fits your skin type or individual preference (see previous recipe). Following are the recommended blending proportions:

Dry skin: 1 part Queen of Hungary Water to 4 parts floral water

Normal skin: 1 part Queen of Hungary Water to 2 parts floral water

Oily skin: 1 part Queen of Hungary Water to 1 part floral water

CHAPTER 17
Herbal Massage

Touch is an important component of good health. We all need to be touched. Many health practitioners now recommend at least one massage per month. Unfortunately, though, some of us may have been touched inappropriately as children so that as adults we find it hard to trust others enough to let them touch us. Perhaps equally tragic are the children who were never touched as babies, and grow up unable to receive loving touch. Please do lovingly touch your children and if you relate to any of the above, get the help you need to heal your past. We all deserve and need to be touched regularly.

TYPES OF MASSAGE

There are a variety of massage practices, but they may not all be styles that you enjoy. How do you choose the massage that is right for you? I think one of the easiest ways to end up happy with the massage you select is to evaluate yourself on a masculinity/femininity scale.

The more feminine, or yin, you are, the gentler your massage should be. The more masculine, or yang, you are, the more you'll appreciate a deeper, more vigorous massage. This is true for both men and women, because both men and women have yin and yang aspects to their being. I think of myself as leaning toward the feminine, and I hate a vigorous massage. It hurts me. My husband likes the opposite. One problem is that most of us give someone the type of massage we like to receive. Don't hesitate to tell your masseuse what you like, and to remind her as often as you need to. It's important that you receive the kind of massage you will enjoy most.

There are many different techniques and styles of massage. For more information, look for a mini-course on massage at your local adult education center. It's worth exploring all the options.

This chapter offers many easy formulas for creating oils that can be used with different massage techniques: herbal infused oils, aromatherapy oils, and a combination of the two. A cream lotion and a moisturizing cream recipe are also included if you want to get a little fancier. The budget-conscious consumer can save a bundle by making her own blended herbal oils.

MASSAGE OILS AND LOTIONS

Massage often is done with straight vegetable oil. That's fine, especially for you minimalists out there. The next step up are aromatherapy oils, which are easy to make and offer the healing elements of both the herbs and their aroma. Herbal infused oils are a bit more work, but they offer the healing elements of the herbs you choose to infuse. You can also create a product with both if you want to get really fancy: Infuse the oil with herbs, then scent with a complementary essential oil.

Care and Storage of Oils

Oils are delicate. Light and heat destabilize them; protect your oils from both. Destabilized oils become rancid. Rancid oils are linked to cancer, so it is important to heed safeguards in making, using, and storing products with oils. Dark amber and cobalt blue bottles afford the most protection from light.

Unfortunately, even the oils purchased at health food stores are rarely packaged in dark containers, with the exception of olive oil, which is the least light sensitive. If you can, purchase oils in bulk from a supplier who has them in a dark container. If you've purchased oil in a clear glass container, either transfer it to a darker bottle or tape brown paper around the glass.

People who live in hot climates may need to refrigerate oil products for most of the year. Those in cooler climates may be

WHY USE NATURAL OILS?

Synthetic oils, petroleum products, and mineral oils create a barrier on the skin. This may seem helpful, but they do not allow the skin to breathe. Vegetable oils are closer to natural human oils and are better for people. Use the petroleum products on your car! Unfortunately, most commercial cosmetics contain mineral or synthetic oils. And if you go for a massage, a budget-conscious masseuse may also be using these products. Ask for a natural vegetable oil. And certainly do not skimp at home, either. (Familiarize yourself with the oils listed on pages 327–329.)

able to get away with storing them in a cool, dark basement. Make small quantities, and refrigerate products that you have heated to make if you are not using them daily.

Aromatherapy Scented Oils

Use pure essential oils rather than synthetic fragrance oils: That way you'll get the full therapeutic value of the scent. Choose the oils that call to you. I don't like to make things too fussy, so I usually choose the simplest method: one scent combined with one main oil, an antioxidant oil, and a few drops of vitamin E oil. But please don't let me stifle your imagination if you want to create blends. Blends are usually made with a top-note essential oil, a middle note, and a base note (see pages 182–183).

SIMPLE LAVENDER OIL

⅔ cup (160 ml) grape-seed oil

⅓ cup (80 ml) wheat germ oil

10 drops vitamin E oil

6 drops lavender essential oil

Yield: 8 ounces

To make:
1. Pour all ingredients into a dark bottle that has a spout.
2. Shake well.

To use:
1. Shake well before each use.
2. Pour the oil into your hands to warm before putting it on the body.
3. Massage into your body using a circular motion.

RED ROSE OIL

2/3 cup (160 ml) grape-
seed oil
1 teaspoon (5 ml)
alkanet root
1/3 cup (80 ml) wheat
germ oil
10 drops vitamin E oil
6 drops rose essen-
tial oil

Yield: 8 ounces

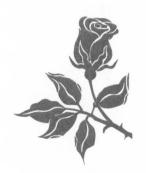

To make:

1. Pour the grapeseed oil and the alkanet root into the top of a double boiler.

2. Gently heat the water bath of the double boiler on the lowest heat.

3. Once the desired degree of redness is achieved in the oil, remove from heat and strain out the alkanet.

4. Add the wheat germ oil, vitamin E, and essential oil to the red oil.

5. Pour all ingredients into a dark bottle that has a spout.

6. Shake well.

To use:

1. Shake well before each use.

2. Pour the oil into your hands to warm before putting it on the body.

3. Massage into your body using a circular motion.

CREAMY LOTION

This wonderful lotion is my adaptation of a Rosemary Gladstar recipe.

2 tablespoons (30 ml) fresh chamomile flowers

2 tablespoons (30 ml) fresh rose buds

2 tablespoons (30 ml) fresh comfrey

2 tablespoons (30 ml) fresh lavender

2 tablespoons (30 ml) fresh calendula

2 fresh sage leaves

1 sprig fresh rosemary

2 tablespoons (30 ml) dried witch hazel bark

2 tablespoons (30 ml) fresh lemon balm

1¼ cups (310 ml) apricot kernel, almond, or grapeseed oil

¼ cup (60 ml) cocoa butter

⅔ cup (180 ml) coconut oil

5 drops essential oil (optional)

1 sterilized, 12-ounce (340-gram) wide-mouthed jar

Yield: Approximately 12 ounces (340 g)

To make:

1. Harvest fresh herbs in midmorning, if possible.

2. Place herbs on paper towels and allow to wilt overnight.

3. Fill jar with wilted herbs.

4. Completely cover the herbs with apricot oil.

5. Each day for the next week, poke herbs down into the oil to release any captured gases. For the three following weeks, do this once a week.

6. After 4 weeks, strain the herbs from the oil.

7. To the infused oil, add cocoa butter and coconut oil. Warm until all ingredients melt together. Scent with the essential oil of your choice.

To use:

1. Pour oil into the palm of your hands to warm.

2. Gently massage into the skin.

MOISTURIZING CREAM MASSAGE

If you prefer to use a moisturizing cream for massage, see the recipes for Rose Pink Face Moisturizer, Lavender Blue Face Moisturizer, and Orange Blossom Face Cream found on pages 250–252.

BASIC MASSAGE STROKES FOR REVITALIZATION

There are many different types of massage and therapeutic touch, and plenty of good books on the subject. Here I offer a simple explanation of a few beginning strokes you can do at home that are quite beneficial.

EFFLEURAGE

This is a gliding stroke over the surface of the skin, usually done with oil or a massage cream. Massage normally starts with light effleurage to gently connect with the person, soothing their nervous system. Gradually, deeper strokes with more pressure may be applied to increase the circulation of blood and lymph.

PETRISSAGE

This kneading movement lifts, presses, and rolls muscle tissue away from the bone to increase circulation of blood and lymph and to detoxify the muscles.

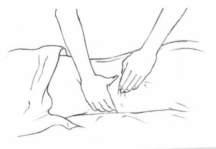

BEGIN WITH GENTLE STROKES

I do not believe in "no pain, no gain." While some sports massage therapists might argue for deep and penetrating massage, rubbing, or scrubbing, I think it is always best to start out gently. A light massage can be quite helpful. It also gives you a chance to identify sensitive areas and pressure preferences, whether you are applying the massage to yourself or to someone else. I urge you to use gentle and loving touch. It makes a big difference. And do ask to be told if you are hurting your "client."

COMPRESSION

Compression is direct pressure to the body and affects muscular, nervous, and energy systems. This technique is done with the thumbs, the whole hand, and even the elbows.

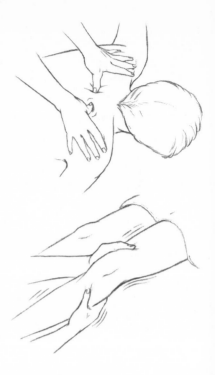

ROCKING

Rocking is a smooth, rhythmic motion that soothes the nervous system. Gently shaking the limbs or rocking parts of the torso encourages the receiver to let go of tension.

DOING MASSAGE AT HOME

In doing massage at home, it is assumed that you have a relationship with the individual you are touching. Most states require a license for massages done for pay. You should be aware of any health conditions of the person you are working on; ask the person if you are not. It can be quite helpful, especially for repeat treatments, to note where a person experiences pain or blockages. Monthly massage can help to alleviate pain and improve circulation.

Getting Ready

Preparation is essential in creating a quality massage experience. Select a place of solitude where you won't be interrupted. A massage table adjusted for your height is ideal, but cushioning a long table or even using a bed or sofa can also be effective. Set up the table so that you can get around all sides, if possible. Make up the table or bed with both a bottom and a top sheet.

Another important factor is warmth. Warmth helps the muscles relax and is essential to a good massage. When lying in the prone position, the body tends to lose heat. Oil on the skin results in it becoming easily chilled. Make sure the room is warm when you start; bring in a space heater if necessary. Also use blankets as needed. Select music that is soothing and pleasing to your "client."

STEP-BY-STEP MASSAGE

This is a simple technique. You may want to learn other massage techniques through your local adult education center. Better yet, take the course with your partner.

◆ Top and bottom sheets
◆ Pillow
◆ Blanket or two
◆ Massage lotion, oil, or cream
◆ Bowl
◆ Relaxing music
◆ Space heater

1. Wash your hands thoroughly before the massage and trim fingernails if necessary.
2. Pour 4 ounces (100 g) of oil into the bowl to start for easy access.
3. Oil your hands and rub them together to warm the oil.
4. Start with your "client" lying face up with his or her body covered by a sheet (and blanket, if needed). Apply the oil to the throat using gentle side-to-side strokes (see page 241 for illustration of facial strokes).
5. Gently swipe across the chin, above the lips, and then across the forehead.
6. Using the fingertips, gently massage in upward strokes, starting at the jaw outside the mouth, coming up along the side of the nose, then across the bridge of the nose.
7. Make several spiraling, circular motions spanning the entire forehead, ending up above and outside the eyes.
8. Press the cheekbones using slight pressure from the outside to inside.
9. Use a spiral, circular stroke on the cheeks.

10. Press along the sides of the neck, working outward to the shoulders.

11. Massage the crown of the head using the fingertips. Press gently, working down and around to the back of the skull.

12. Uncover one arm, leaving the rest of the body draped. Gently holding the wrist, shake the arm from side to side. With both hands around the arm, gently squeeze, working back and forth starting at the shoulder and working down to the hand.

13. Do the same on the other arm and then each leg.

14. Have the "client" turn over, and work on the back. Starting at the base of the spine, gently push on the spine, working up to the top of the shoulders. Rub the shoulders and top of the back all over.

Privacy

Creating a space where you will not be disturbed is essential. Let your husband, housemates, or kids know that you are going to be off-limits for a while. Let them know how long you need. Put up a "Do not disturb" sign. Enlist your family's cooperation. Before you start your treatment, take the phone off the hook or put on the answering machine.

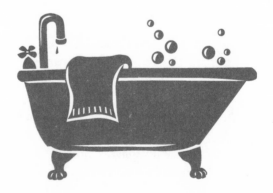

CREATING AROMATHERAPY

There are many ways to scent your home using essential oils. Check out your local health food store or perfume shop to learn about diffuser styles. Some diffusers require a tea light or votive candle, other are ceramic rings that can be placed over a lightbulb: The heat of the candle or bulb releases the scent. I prefer the candle over the electric choices.

For a lighter scent, small aromatic pottery works well. These small, bottle-shaped pieces of pottery are left partially unglazed. You simply uncork and add some essential oil. The essential oil seeps through the unglazed pottery and cork. This also works well for scenting your car.

The least expensive way to scent your home is to gently simmer herbs in a saucepan with water. Toss a handful of dried or two handfuls of fresh aromatic herbs in a saucepan full of boiling water, lower to simmer, and voilá! All the mints and aromatics work well with this technique, including lavender, rose, lovage, marjoram, sage, oregano, and thyme. Spices are also wonderfully effective, and you only need about a 1/4 cup. Cloves, cinnamon chips, aniseed and fennel seeds, bay leaf, and nutmeg can be used in combination or alone. If you are going to use the stove, you might want to create a floral water at the same time (see pages 253–254).

CHAPTER 18
Herbal Body Wraps and Skin Treatments

Body wraps and herbal skin treatments are designed to increase circulation, remove toxins, and promote smooth, soft, supple skin. The skin is the body's largest organ of elimination. Good circulation to the skin helps rid the body of harmful substances and enhances secretion of natural oils, which moisturize the skin and keep the body healthy. Blood flowing to the skin brings oxygen to the surface; blood and lymph flowing away from the skin release and eliminate toxins. By stimulating circulation, the body is better able to eliminate impurities.

Over the centuries, various cultures have developed techniques to enhance circulation and produce healthy, glowing skin. Most of these involve creating friction on the skin, or exfoliating, a process that assists the blood and lymph systems in releasing wastes. Ayurveda uses a silk-mitt exfoliation technique. Romans used dry brushing. And seafaring cultures have used sea salt, seaweed, and the sun for increasing circulation.

Many of these time-tested techniques are featured at today's most elegant spas. In this chapter, you will learn how you can practice them at home. I also show you how you can prepare and apply luxurious herb, fruit, and vegetable body scrubs, wraps, and masks, along with thalassotherapy, to create pampering and nurturing sessions at your own home spa.

> **CAUTION**
>
> The treatments presented in this chapter are beneficial for addressing a wide range of health concerns. However, consult your doctor before engaging in the treatments, especially if you have varicose veins or circulation or heart problems.

THE BENEFITS OF INCREASED CIRCULATION

Most of us have sluggish skin and don't realize it. You may have heard the saying, "Animals sweat, men perspire, and women merely glow." In truth, it would be better if we were more like animals on this account. The inability to sweat all over, especially when exercising or in a sauna, is a symptom of poor skin elimination due to poor circulation. Dull complexion, cold hands and feet, and constipation are other signs of poor circulation. The treatments in this chapter alleviate these conditions by increasing circulation, bringing warmth to the extremities, improving the complexion, and acting as a mild laxative. Thus, no need to feel that you're being overindulgent with these treatments — they are part of staying healthy and feeling well!

Weight Control and Cellulite

Unwelcome weight gain and cellulite can also often be managed by increasing blood circulation to the skin on a daily basis. Good circulation is not just a surface phenomenon; it makes for healthier internal organs as well. Healthy organ functioning aids metabolism and weight management.

Weight gain sometimes can be remedied or controlled by raising your activity level, which in turn increases circulation. The sluggishness of weight gain may show up in the skin as dullness or pallor. Increasing circulation helps let go of the pounds and in turn creates more vibrant, alive skin — and the healthy glow that goes along with it.

DANGERS OF OVERUSING SOAP AND MOISTURIZERS

Two everyday hygiene practices that inhibit circulation and block the skin surface are excessive use of soap and overuse of moisturizing creams, especially those containing petroleum products. While Americans are often surprised at the European practice of bathing less frequently, we are actually the ones who are caught up in a "hygiene paranoia." Manufacturers of hygiene products play on these fears of being "stinky" or in some way unattractive with the heavy emphasis on deodorizing in their advertisements.

Regardless, our practice of washing all of our body with soap is unnecessary

MINIMIZE USE OF MOISTURIZING CREAM

Body moisturizing creams should be applied lightly and sparingly. By increasing the use of the circulation-enhancing techniques suggested in this chapter, you can gradually diminish your dependence on moisture creams. As a result of exfoliation, the natural oils in your skin will come to the surface to create a baby-bottom softness without any added cream.

and can even be detrimental to good circulation, not to mention costly. Don't fret if you love good soaps; they certainly have their place. Soaps are meant for the hairy parts of the body, that is, the hair, underarms, and pubic region. Soaps are okay for sweaty and dirty areas as well, such as under the breasts, your hands and feet, or other parts that may get dirty as a result of your daily work. Other parts of your body, however, even if you are a man with a lot of hair on your back, are best washed simply with water or possibly a slightly acid rinse of water and vinegar or lemon juice.

The natural pH of the skin is slightly acidic. By constantly putting basic (as opposed to acidic) products such as soap on the skin, it is constantly fighting to get back to its natural pH. The result is dry, itchy skin, and the need for moisture creams.

Moisture creams, unfortunately, also inhibit the skin's natural functions. Most of the commercial products available contain petroleum-based ingredients that block the natural breathing of the skin and inhibit circulation. Creams with purer ingredients, however, may be very expensive. You can save both your money and your skin by making your own moisture creams. The recipes in chapter 16 (see pages 235–237) for the face and neck are inexpensive enough to use all over your body.

A WARNING FOR ITCHY-SKIN SUFFERERS

If you have itchy skin, be especially careful to avoid using soap excessively, bathing in a tub full of soapsuds, and over-moisturizing your skin. All of these practices interfere with your skin's ability to maintain its natural pH. Your itching may clear up by omitting soap or by bathing in or rinsing with a combination of water and vinegar or lemon juice.

EXFOLIATION TECHNIQUES

Exfoliating the skin is a process by which you use an abrasive surface to rub the skin (usually before showering), scraping away any dead cells on your skin's surface, increasing circulation, and making the skin glow. If you have delicate skin, please don't give up on exfoliation. Start out gently and in no time you'll be able to tolerate more vigorous scrubs and rubs. Don't be alarmed if you start to notice a few blemishes; this is normal as the skin starts to slough off impurities, and it will diminish as your skin gets healthier.

LOOFAH SPONGE RUB

You will find a variety of loofah products in the health and beauty aisle of many drugstores. Experiment with using whole loofahs, sewing a piece into a washcloth to create a mitt, or making a disk of the softer part for your face.

Materials needed: Loofah sponge, style of your choice.
To use: Wet the loofah in the shower and rub it all over your body to invigorate the skin. You can also use it to slough off dry skin before showering. Standing in the tub, rub the loofah over your dry body in a circular motion, starting at the extremities and working toward the torso.

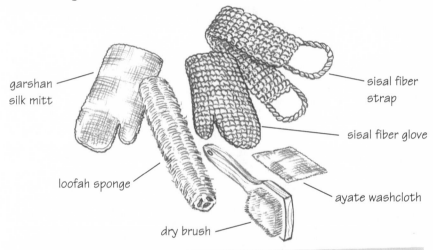

garshan silk mitt

sisal fiber strap

sisal fiber glove

loofah sponge

ayate washcloth

dry brush

GROWING LOOFAH

The loofah sponge is not a sponge at all — it's a plant (part of the cucumber family) that you can grow in your garden. You may be able to obtain seeds from a purchased loofah; shake it and see if any fall out. If not, you can purchase loofah seeds at most garden centers. The seeds are slow to germinate, so start them indoors and transplant them out later. The plants enjoy growing on a trellis for support and take about 75 days to produce gourds. When the skin turns brown, it is time to harvest. Dry the gourds, then soak them in water until the outer skin disappears, and you've got your exfoliating sponge. These make great gifts, too.

ROMAN DRY BRUSHING

The stiffer the bristles on your brush, the better the lymphatic stimulation you'll generate. If you have trouble finding a dry brush at your local natural food or health store, see Resources on pages 336–338.

Materials needed: Natural bristle brush (palm-size; also available with optional stick for use on back).

To use: Standing in the bathtub (to catch the falling skin), brush the dry skin all over your body, starting with the fingertips and arms and working inward toward the torso. Next, brush your legs and move upward toward the torso. Some areas may be more sensitive than others, for instance, the breasts and neck, yet the treatment is quite good for them as well. The more often you do this treatment, the less sensitive your skin will become. Once or twice a day is recommended.

RECOMMENDED EXFOLIATING TECHNIQUES

It's important to brush or rub your body in the particular sequence that is most conducive to circulation. Begin by rubbing the extremities (arms and legs) and working inward to the torso. This encourages the blood flow in toward the heart. Then, rub your torso to encourage the blood to flow out from the heart through the organs and to the entire body.

These exfoliation techniques can be used on all parts of the body except the face. Gradually, as you use these techniques more and more, you will find that your skin tolerates a more vigorous scrub or rub. But be careful not to get carried away and rub or brush your skin to the point of bleeding. If you are like me and tend to have itchy skin, the brushing and rubbing may feel so good that you overdo it. One way to treat the itchiness is to take regular vinegar baths (see page 290).

GARSHAN SILK-MITT TREATMENT

This exfoliation technique comes from the Ayurvedic healing techniques developed in India to create vigor, energy, and balance in the body, mind, emotions, and beyond. If you know someone with rough hands you won't need the mitt — just talk that person into giving you a rub with his or her bare hands.

Materials needed: ¼ yard (23 cm) raw silk, needle and thread (or sewing machine). Makes 1 mitt.

To make: Cut two mitten-shaped pieces from the raw silk. With right sides together, sew a ⅝" seam around the mitt, leaving the bottom open. Turn the mitt right side out.

To use: With the mitt on your hand, scrub your entire body, wet or dry, starting from the extremities and moving inward toward the torso. This is good preparation for the cellulite body wrap.

AYATE FIBER CLOTH RUB

The century plant grows in the Southwest and Mexico and has been used for centuries by Native peoples for exfoliating. Look for products made from ayate or agave in a health food store. The loosely woven cloth shrinks to a finer weave when it is put in water.

To use: Wet the ayate cloth and rub it over your entire body when taking a shower or bath, starting from the extremities and moving inward to the torso.

SISAL FIBER RUB

Similar to the ayate fiber cloth, sisal fiber cloth is often made into gloves and back straps for rubbing on the body. Look for these products in your local health food store (or see Resources).

To use: Wet the sisal fiber glove or strap and rub over entire body when showering or bathing, working from the extremities inward. The glove is especially good for rubbing on fleshy areas such as the thighs.

HERBAL BODY SCRUBS

Another way to exfoliate the skin and remove toxins is to make a grainy herbal body scrub. Any number of fruits, grains, herbs, minerals, and vegetables can been used alone or in combination to make scrubs. Most substances that are safe to eat are also safe to use on the skin, provided you do not have an allergy. Several recipes for herbal body scrubs follow, but please don't limit yourself to these combinations. You can really let your imagination run wild: Mix up your own concoctions, based on the ingredients you happen to have on hand or your favorite fruits, herbs, and vegetables. When you're experimenting, try making small batches before you go to full-scale production.

AVOCADO MOISTURE SCRUB

Tired of sprouting or just throwing away avocado pits? Here's a great way to use them, and it gives you low-fat dieters an excuse to splurge. Avocado, high in fat and oil, is very therapeutic for dry skin.

2–3 fresh avocado pits
1 cup (250 ml) milk, water, or yogurt

Yield: 1 treatment

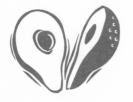

To make:

1. Let the avocado pits dry for a few days, but not to the point of becoming rock hard (or they will break your spice mill).

2. Using a spice mill or coffee grinder, grind the dried avocado pits to create a grainy, mealy powder.

3. Add the water, milk, or yogurt to the powder and mix to form a paste.

To use:

1. Sitting or standing in the bathtub or shower, pat avocado paste all over your body using a circular motion. Start from the tips of the extremities and work toward the torso. Don't forget to apply this mixture to your face, too.

2. Leave on for 10 minutes, then shower, first with warm water, then cooler water.

3. Pat dry.

OATMEAL ALMOND BODY SCRUB

Many ground nuts make excellent scrubs: With their high fat content, they moisturize while exfoliating. Oatmeal is quite moisturizing, making this recipe especially good for dry or itchy skin. Be sure to tie up your hair or wear a shower cap, as this can get messy.

1 cup (250 ml) oatmeal
½ cup (125 ml) almonds
½ cup (125 ml) dried rose petals
½ cup (125 ml) dried lemon balm
1 cup (250 ml) white cosmetic clay
½ cup (125 ml) yogurt
Juice of 1 lemon

Yield: 1 treatment

To make:

1. Grind or powder the oatmeal, almonds, rose petals, and lemon balm separately using a spice mill or blender, leaving some grit in each.

2. In a large bowl, mix all the dry ingredients with a wire whisk.

3. Add the lemon juice and yogurt and blend thoroughly.

4. Add water as needed.

To use:

1. Sitting in the bathtub, slather on the scrub. Using a circular motion, start with the toes and work up the leg.

2. Next work on the arms, starting with the hands and working toward the torso.

3. Using a circular motion, massage in the mix to the torso.

4. Sit in the tub for 10 minutes, allowing the clay mix to dry on the skin.

5. Shower or bathe in warm water, gently rinsing the skin.

6. Pat dry.

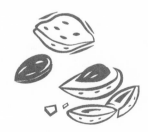

HERBAL BODY MASKS AND POLISHES

Body masks, designed to moisturize the skin, use ingredients with emollient, humectant, nourishing, and healing properties. As with the body scrubs, the masks use the fleshier parts of fruits, herbs, vegetables, dairy products, and oils. These treatments are similar to those offered in some of the more fabulous spas. Don't be afraid to use these as a springboard for developing your own personalized recipes.

APPLE PULP POMADE

Especially good for those with sensitive skin, this recipe is great to make at the height of apple season.

15 medium-size apples (McIntosh work well)

½ cup (125 ml) apricot kernel oil

1 tablespoon (15 ml) lemon zest

Yield: 1 treatment

To make:

1. Cut up apples and put in a large pot.
2. Add a little water, as needed.
3. Simmer and mash till the mixture is the consistency of applesauce, approximately 30 minutes.
4. Pour off excess water.
5. Add apricot kernel oil and lemon zest; mix well. Use while still warm.

To use:

1. While sitting in the tub or shower, slather the warm apple mixture all over your body, and hair, too, if you like.
2. Rest in the tub with the mixture on for 10 minutes.
3. Shower in warm water.
4. Pat dry.

CUCUMBER BODY PIZZA

Don't have the time or the inclination for mixing lotions and potions today? Are you suffering from the "itches" or poison ivy? Try this Cucumber Body Pizza. It is cooling, draws out the itch, and isn't messy. You may want to have a partner around to apply the cucumber slices for you.

3–5 cucumbers

Yield: 1 treatment

To make:

1. Thinly slice the cucumbers and place on a plate.

To use:

1. Lie face down in a comfortable position in a warm place. Have a friend place cucumber slices all over the back side of your body, so they are just touching but not overlapping. Use about half the total slices.

2. Rest quietly for 10 to 20 minutes to allow the cucumber slices and juice to penetrate your skin.

3. Remove the slices.

4. Turn over and apply the rest of the slices to your front side. Relax for 10 to 20 minutes. You may want to shower afterwards, but it is best not to for at least 4 hours, as the cucumber will continue to work on the skin during that time

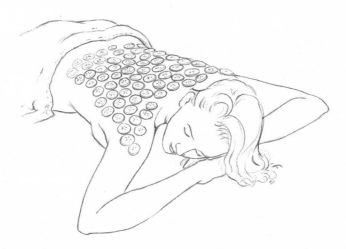

SALT GLOW

The Salt Glow is a vigorous circulatory stimulant that removes dead surface cells and dirt, leaving your skin soft and gleaming. Salt Glow stimulates the secretion of your natural skin oils and is especially helpful for sluggish skin. You may fear being dried out with this rub, but I find my moderately dry skin loves this treatment, and leaves me feeling like a baby's bottom all over. The salts encourage the skin to secrete its natural oils.

2   cups (500 ml)
    coarse sea salt
¼   cup (50 ml) water

Yield: 1 treatment

To use:

1. Place the salt in a bowl and wet it with the water.

2. Fill the tub ankle-deep with warm water and step into the tub.

3. Starting with your arms, wet them and then rub the salt vigorously on the skin, moving from the fingertips to shoulders until the skin is aglow.

4. Next wet your legs. Now rub on the salt, beginning at your feet and moving up to your thighs.

5. Next, wet the torso and then rub on the salt in a circular motion.

6. Once your whole body has been rubbed, sit in the warm tub of water to relax, allowing the salt to work on your skin while sitting in the ankle-deep water for a few minutes.

7. Rinse with warm water and follow with a cool rinse.

Variations:

◆ Substitute ½ cup (125 ml) grapeseed oil (or almond, apricot kernel, or olive oil) for the ¼ cup (60 ml) water.

◆ Add 6 to 8 drops of essential oil to the straight salt or salt and oil mix.

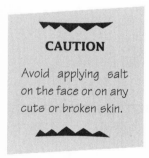

CAUTION

Avoid applying salt on the face or on any cuts or broken skin.

AROMATHERAPY BATH SALTS

Each pure essential oil has a scent and character all its own. Select one for your Salt Glow that has the therapeutic benefits to suit your needs and mood. Here are a few of the more common ones you might want to try, along with their benefits. For more information about aromatherapy, See Part II.

- ◆ **Chamomile:** relaxing and calming
- ◆ **Clary Sage:** warming; promotes feelings of well-being
- ◆ **Basil:** relieves mental fatigue and nervousness
- ◆ **Eucalyptus:** promotes clear breathing
- ◆ **Jasmine:** antidepressant; supports feelings of confidence
- ◆ **Lavender:** soothing
- ◆ **Orange:** cheering
- ◆ **Peppermint:** stimulating, increases energy
- ◆ **Pine:** alleviates fatigue

PUMPKIN SLATHER

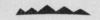

Like so many of the squash vegetables, pumpkins are excellent moisturizers for your body.

1 small pumpkin
1 cup (250 ml) yogurt
Juice from 1 lemon

Yield: 1 treatment

To make:

1. Cut up the pumpkin, removing skin and scooping out pulp. Place the flesh in a pot with a small amount of water.

2. Cook the pumpkin until mashable with a potato masher.

3. Remove from heat, mash pumpkin, and add yogurt and lemon juice. Use while still warm.

To use:

1. Sit in the tub or shower, and slather the warm pumpkin mixture all over your dry body, and hair, too, if you like.

2. Rest in the tub with the mixture on your body for 10 minutes.

3. Shower in warm water.

4. Pat dry.

HERBAL BODY WRAPS

In spas the world over, clients pay big bucks for these treatments. Wraps are credited with creating all kinds of miracles, including weight loss and cellulite removal. Regardless of whether these claims are true, this is a great way to be pampered. You may need to recruit assistance with the wrapping part of this treatment. What a great Valentine's Day ritual for you to share with a partner.

BASIC HERBAL WRAP FORMULA

2 cups (500 ml) fresh herbs (1 cup [250 ml] dried)

1 large cotton sheet ripped into 2-inch-wide (5-cm) strips, each as long as possible

Clean plastic drop cloth or tarp

Large basin or spaghetti pot

Yield: 1 treatment

To make:

1. Place the herbs in the basin or pot.

2. Pour boiling water over the herbs and cover. Let steep for 5 minutes.

3. Remove as many herbs as you can from the pot using a strainer.

4. Add the sheet strips to the pot and steep for 5 more minutes.

To use:

1. Exfoliate using your preferred method, then shower before using this treatment.

2. Lay the drop cloth or tarp on a comfortable recliner, chair, or bed — preferably in a warm room.

SUGGESTED HERBS FOR USE IN A BODY WRAP

For stimulation and energy: peppermint, rosemary, juniper, lemon peel

For relaxation: lavender, clary sage, chamomile, tangerine peel

For healing and antiseptic properties: calendula, eucalyptus, tea tree, lavender

For aches and pains: 1 cup (250 ml) Epsom salts plus rosemary, lavender, or eucalyptus

For itchy skin: red clover plus 1 cup (250 ml) apple cider vinegar or lemon juice

3. Remove the sheet strips one by one, wringing out the liquid. Wrap each strip around your body snugly. Start with the arms, then follow with the legs, the torso, and the head.

4. Once all the strips are wrapped and the body is covered, sit in the chair and wrap the drop cloth or tarp around your body.

5. Cover yourself with a few blankets and relax quietly for 10 minutes.

6. Unwrap the strips from your body and slowly emerge from your cocoon.

7. It is best not to shower for at least 4 hours afterwards and preferably not for 24 hours.

WRAPPING TECHNIQUES

Strips should overlap each other, so that each part of the body is covered twice. When coming to the end of a strip, tuck it under a wrapped area near it, keeping the strip snug but not too tight.

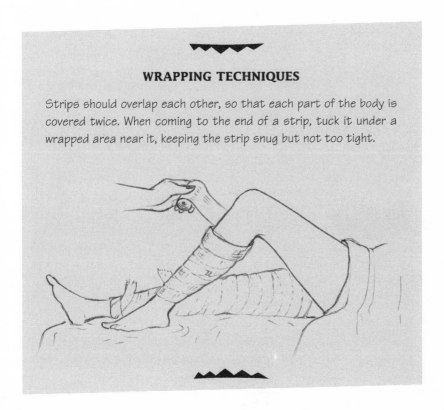

CELLULITE BODY WRAP

This body wrap is aimed at reducing those little cottage cheese bumps that occur on many women's derrieres and thighs. It is most effective when done in a warm room. You may need to enlist some help with wrapping the cellophane.

8 drops of grapefruit essential oil
2 drops each of essential oils of thyme, fennel, lavender, geranium, juniper berry
2 cups (500 ml) almond oil
Cellophane wrap

Yield: 1 treatment

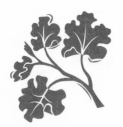

To use:

1. Turn up the heat in the bathroom or bedroom.

2. In a plastic squirt bottle, combine the essential oils with the almond oil, shaking well.

3. Exfoliate the skin using your preferred method (loofah, silk mitt, dry brush, or ayate or sisal fiber — see pages 269–271).

4. While standing in the shower or bathtub or on a towel in your bedroom, knead the oil mixture generously into the skin on your arms, legs, and torso, avoiding the face and neck.

5. Encase your legs in cellophane beginning at the toes and working up to the thighs. I have found it easier to apply the cellophane when the whole cellophane roll is cut in half or thirds to 2-inch (5-cm) widths. Wrap snugly, but don't cut off the circulation.

6. Wrap your arms, beginning at the hands and moving up to the upper arms. Complete by wrapping the torso.

7. Relax in a warm room for 20 minutes. You can make the tub as comfy as possible with a pillow for your head, or sit on a comfortable chair or bed that you've covered with a towel.

8. Remove the cellophane wrap from your body; shower first with warm water, then with cooler water.

9. Pat skin dry.

BASIC CLAY BODY WRAP FORMULA

Use this French clay body wrap at least once a month to remove toxins from the body and leave the skin soft and smooth.

½ cup (125 ml) dried herbs

1 cup (250 ml) distilled water

1 cup (250 ml) French, green, or red clay

1 tablespoon (15 ml) almond or apricot kernel oil

1 tablespoon (15 ml) yogurt

3 drops essential oil of your choice

2 large bedsheets torn into 6-inch-wide (15-cm) strips, each as long as possible

1 large pot of boiling water

New medium-size paintbrush

Yield: 1 treatment

To make:

1. Place the herbs in a clean, 10-ounce (284-gram) glass jar.

2. Bring the distilled water to a boil.

3. Pour the boiling water over the herbs, cover, and allow to steep for 10 minutes to make an herbal infusion.

4. Put the clay in a medium-size bowl; add the almond oil and yogurt and mix.

5. Add the herbal infusion to the clay mixture, herbs and all.

6. Add the bedsheet strips to the large pot of boiling water.

To use:

1. Bring the clay mixture and the pot with strips to the bathroom.

2. Standing in the bathtub, begin applying the clay mixture to your legs with the paintbrush, starting at the toes and working up to the thighs.

3. Wring out one of the fabric strips and begin wrapping your legs from the toes up. Continue to wrap snugly (but not cutting off the circulation), using more strips as needed.

4. Repeat step 3 for your arms, starting with the fingertips and working up to the shoulders.

5. Apply clay to torso and wrap, as in step 3.

6. Relax in the tub for 10 to 20 minutes.

7. Unwrap your body and shower with tepid water.

8. Pat dry.

HOT AND COLD STIMULATION

You may know about the Scandinavian practice of sitting in a warm sauna and then going out to jump in the snow. This combination of hot and cold body immersions is good for the circulation and is a great way to stay warm in winter. Most people cringe at the suggestion of taking a cold-water shower, especially in winter. But listen up, all you undershirt, turtleneck, and sweater people who are cold all winter: This is your cure.

Consider how chilled you usually feel when stepping out of a warm shower into the cooler air of your home. You can avoid this chilling sensation by showering first with warm water and then with cold water, which stimulates your circulation. After this shocking treatment, when you step out of the shower, your body responds immediately by bringing more blood to the surface and creating warmth, since the last sensation you felt in the shower was colder than the air outside it. Your body is warming up, rather than chilling down!

Hot and Cold Stimulating Shower

1. Shower as usual.
2. Before the shower is over, turn the water to the coldest temperature you can stand for 15 seconds, exposing all your body parts to the water, especially the nape of the neck.
3. Turn the water to the hottest you can stand for 15 seconds, again exposing all parts to the water. Note: Be sure you have a scald guard on your faucet, or that the temperature of the water does not exceed 110°F.
4. Turn the water back to the coldest you can tolerate for another 15 seconds. (Screaming and shouting are optional!)
5. Turn off the water. Towel dry, and notice how warm you feel.

THALASSOTHERAPY

Thalassotherapy is a Greek word used to refer to spa treatments that employ seawater and seaweed. Perhaps you think of salty seawater as drying, but these treatments are actually wonderful for dry skin and cellulite. Seaweed also increases circulation, thus helping to firm the skin and reduce fat accumulation.

SEAWEED BODY WRAP

You may need some help wrapping the gauze around your body for this treatment. When you're finished, the gauze can be rinsed and laundered and then used again.

2 cups (500 ml) clay of your choice
½ cup (125 ml) kelp powder
½ cup (125 ml) dulse powder
Juice from 1 lemon, divided in two
1 cup (250 ml) hot to warm water, divided in two
Enough gauze to cover your body
2 or 3 large beach towels

Yield: 1 treatment

To make:

1. In a large bowl, mix together the clay and seaweed powders with a wire whisk.

2. Place half the mixture in another bowl, then add the juice of ½ lemon and ½ cup hot to warm water, mixing to form a paste (reserve the rest of the lemon juice and water to add to the rest of the mixture when you need it).

To use:

1. Prepare your skin for the treatment first by dry brushing or exfoliating with another method of your choice (see pages 268–271).

2. Crank up the heat in the bathroom if possible, or bring in a space heater.

3. Standing in the bathtub or shower, first wet the skin. Then slather the seaweed mix onto your skin, starting with the feet.

4. Start wrapping the gauze firmly in an upward fashion around the clay-seaweed mixture on your body, beginning at the toes and working up the legs. Don't cut off the circulation, but keep it snug.

5. After both legs are covered, work from your fingers up your arms. When you run out of the mixture, add the juice and water to the other half of the recipe you had set aside.

6. Wrap the torso next, then the hair and neck, avoiding the face.

7. Lie back in the tub, covering yourself with beach towels, and get cozy for 20 minutes.

8. Remove the gauze from your body. Shower with warm water, then with cool water.

9. Pat dry.

CHAPTER 19
Herbal Bathing Rituals

Bathing has long been a favored art for those who cannot resist the lure of calming, cleansing waters. These pleasure seekers are not new to our time but in fact are ancient. Early civilizations developed at the edges of rivers, lakes, and oceans, clearly recognizing the purifying, life-giving essence of water. The sacred use of water is central to many religions: Consider Christian baptism, Islamic preparation for prayer of ablutions, and the Native American sweat lodge, for example.

Bathing is still one of the most important rituals of our time. My bathroom is my sanctuary. I can't think of a more divine daily practice than bathing by candlelight. Water alone is quite pleasant, and being a purist and always looking for the least time-consuming preparations, I appreciate the uncomplicated in life. To enhance the sensory pleasure of the bathing experience, try some of the following simple, yet exotic, ideas. Bath products make wonderful gifts for yourself and for others. I include recipes for a variety of bath crystals, bath bubbles, milk baths, vinegar baths, and steam baths, along with information on how to use compresses and poultices and sitz baths for bathing and healing small areas of your body. (See chapter 20 for hand soaks and footbaths.)

SOAP

If you've ever made soap from scratch, you know it can be great fun but a little messy — and it may be more time-consuming than your schedule allows. (If you haven't tried making soap from scratch and are intrigued, I recommend Susan Miller Cavitch's *The Natural Soap Book*.)

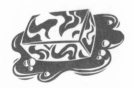

LAVENDER SOAP BALLS

This recipe enables you to create a beautiful product from simple ingredients in just a short time. This is a fun project to do with children, and it's especially good for those who have to be nagged to wash their hands!

2 bars mild, unscented soap (castile or vegetable-based)

½ cup (125 ml) dried lavender blossoms

5 drops essential oil of lavender

¼ cup (60 ml) warm water

Yield: Approximately 12 soap balls

To make:

1. Using a cheese grater, grate the soap bars into a large bowl.

2. Add the lavender to the grated soap.

3. Add the essential oil to the soap mixture, combining thoroughly.

4. Add the warm water and stir.

5. Roll heaping tablespoons of the mix into smooth balls.

6. Place on a cookie sheet and allow to air-dry completely, which will take approximately 2 days.

BATH CRYSTALS

You'll find a variety of herbal and aromatherapy bath crystals at almost any pharmacy, health food emporium, or department store. I usually bring one or two of these prepackaged products to my classes to show students to demystify the "exotic" ingredients on the label. Desert salt sounds pretty extravagant, for instance. How can you obtain it short of taking a trip to the Sahara? How about a stroll down the laundry detergent aisle in your local supermarket? Yes, borax, the 20-mule-team stuff, is actually desert salt. Soda ash is another exotic name for a common household staple — baking soda. Since the beginning of time, individuals have used salts for skin treatments. None of these ingredients costs much. By making your own products you can save money, and at the same time customize the blend to fit your tastes and needs.

FINE CRYSTAL BATHING SAND

You'll see this product packaged in fancy jars or envelopes with a hefty price tag; you can make your own for a fraction of the cost.

2 cups (500 ml) borax (desert salt)

½ cup (125 ml) fine ground sea salt

½ cup (125 ml) baking soda (soda ash)

¼ cup (60 ml) white clay

½ cup (125 ml) dried herb of your choice

10 drops essential oil

Yield: Approximately 3¾ cups (930 ml)

To make:

1. In a large bowl, mix together the salts, baking soda, and clay.

2. Prepare the dried herb by powdering in a spice mill, crumbling by hand, or leaving whole if you prefer (see box below on preparing herbs).

3. Add the dried herbs to the salt mix, stirring with a wire whisk.

4. Scent the mixture using the essential oil of your choice. (Be sure to choose oils that are safe for external use.) Do not overscent; excess oil results in a clumpy, unattractive product — trust me.

5. Mix well with a wire whisk, then cover with a towel.

6. Leave overnight to fix the scent.

7. In the morning, thoroughly mix again and package.

To use:

Add ¼ to ½ cup (60 to 125 ml) sand to a tubful of warm water.

A NOTE ON PREPARING HERBS

Crush the dried herbs for bath sand as finely or coarsely as you like, or you can even leave them whole. Powdering is the best idea for anyone with temperamental plumbing; if you leave the herbs whole, it's probably a good idea to package the finished mixture in a small muslin bag for use in the tub. This will also make tub cleaning easier than if you throw the sand freely into the tub.

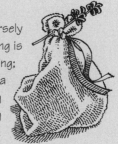

HEALING SALT CRYSTALS

If your health practitioner has recommended Epsom salts baths for your aching bones, this recipe is for you. It is very similar to the Fine Crystal Bathing Sand recipe, but has a coarser texture.

1 cup (250 ml) borax (desert salt)
2 cups (500 ml) Epsom salts
½ cup (125 ml) coarse sea salt
¼ cup (60 ml) baking soda
¼ cup (60 ml) white clay
½ cup (125 ml) dried herb of your choice
10 drops essential oil

Yield: 4 cups (1 liter)

To make:
1. In a large bowl, mix together the borax, salts, baking soda, and clay.
2. Prepare the dried herb by powdering in a spice mill, crumbling by hand, or leaving whole if you prefer (see box on preparing herbs).
3. Add the dried herbs to the salt mix, stirring with a wire whisk.
4. Scent the mix using the essential oil of your choice. (Be sure to choose oils that are safe for external use.) Do not overscent; excess oil will result in a clumpy, unattractive product.
5. Mix well with wire whisk, then cover with a towel.
6. Leave overnight to fix the scent.
7. In the morning, thoroughly mix again and package.
To use:
Add ¼ to ½ cup (60 to 125 ml) sand to a tubful of warm water.

PACKAGING BATH SALTS

Package salts in pretty jars, zipseal bags, muslin bags, or small seed-type envelopes. You can decorate any of these packages with stickers, ribbons or raffia, and bows, or have your children draw pictures on the envelopes before filling.

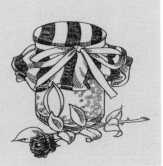

BUBBLE BATHS

Bubble baths are great fun for the kid in all of us. Unfortunately, they can leave your skin dry and itchy. Be sure to rinse thoroughly with clear water when finished bathing. If you are prone to dry, itchy skin, rinse in vinegar or lemon juice combined with water to counter the alkalinity of the soap and return your skin to its more natural pH, which is slightly acidic. The citrus and kiddie bubbles that follow are based on a recipe in Janice Cox's book, *Natural Beauty at Home.*

CITRUS BUBBLES

1 lemon
1 egg white
1 packet unflavored gelatin (¼ ounce [7 g])
1 tablespoon (15 ml) sesame, safflower, or canola oil
¼ cup (60 ml) unscented castile liquid soap
2 drops each lime, lemon, orange, and grapefruit essential oils

Yield: Makes enough bubbles for 1 bath

To make:

1. Juice the lemon and pour into a small container.
2. Lightly beat the egg white in a small bowl.
3. Fold the gelatin into the egg white.
4. In a bowl, combine all ingredients, including the lemon juice, and mix well.

To use:

1. Start running the water for your bath.
2. When the tub is half full of water, pour the Citrus Bubbles into the bath directly under the tap and mix well.
3. Slip into the tub as soon as the mix is poured to receive the full benefit of the aromas from the essential oils.
4. Rinse with cool water after bathing.

KIDDIE BUBBLES

This is a fun recipe for children and has none of the chemicals found in most commercial products.

1 egg white
2 packets unflavored gelatin (½ ounce [14 g])
⅓ cup (80 ml) liquid castile soap
1 tablespoon (15 ml) sesame oil
6 drops essential oil of orange or strawberry

Yield: Makes enough bubbles for 1 bath

To make:
1. Beat the egg white slightly.
2. Fold in the gelatin.
3. Pour all ingredients into a bowl and mix well.

To use:
1. Start running the water for your bath.
2. When the tub is half full of water, pour the Kiddie Bubbles into the bath directly under the tap and mix well.
3. Slip into the tub as soon as the mix is poured to receive the full benefit of the aromas from the essential oils.
4. Rinse with cool water after bathing.

SPICE ISLAND ESCAPE

Can't get away to the Spice Islands in the next week or so? Try this bath oil — it's the next best thing! This recipe is adapted from *The World Beauty Book* by Jessica Harris.

¼ cup (60 ml) sesame oil
⅛ cup (30 ml) cinnamon chips
5 whole cloves
1 large bay leaf, crumbled
Dash nutmeg or mace

Yield: 1 treatment

To make:
1. Place all ingredients in a glass jar. Let them steep for 1 week, shaking daily.
2. Strain the spices out of the oil using a fine mesh strainer.

To use:
1. Start filling the tub with water. When the tub is half full of water, pour the spicy sesame oil under the tap.
2. Slip into the tub as soon as the mix is poured to receive the full benefit of the scented oil.
3. Rinse with cool water after bathing.

VINEGAR HERBAL BATHS

In much the same way as you might make herbal vinegars for your salads, you can also create products that help restore the natural pH of your skin. Vinegar rinses are great diluted after bathing in alkaline soaps. Slightly acid baths are good for itchy skin. Vinegar rinses leave your hair shiny (see chapter 15).

ROSE PETAL VINEGAR BATH

Roses have been used for eons to enhance beauty and as symbols of love. I can't bear to pick my rose petals when the flowers are young; I always wait until the petals are almost ready to fall off naturally. Probably some of the medicinal and aromatic properties of the plant are lost, but they work fine for me and I get to enjoy the flowers longer. Any rose petals will work — wild roses or cultivated varieties — but please don't use your Valentine's Day bouquet, as commercial roses are heavily sprayed with pesticides.

2 cups (500 ml) fresh rose petals

1 quart (1 liter) apple cider vinegar

Yield: 2 baths

To make:
1. Collect fresh rose petals.
2. Spread the rose petals on paper towels and allow them to wilt overnight.
3. Pour vinegar into a saucepan.
4. Bring to a boil on medium heat.
5. Place the rose petals in a sterilized, wide-mouthed jar.
6. Pour the vinegar over the petals.
7. Cap the jar with a nonmetal lid and steep for 2 weeks.
8. Strain and bottle in sterilized vinegar bottles.
9. Cork or cap and decorate with stickers, raffia, and ribbons.

To use:
1. Begin drawing a tub of warm water.
2. When the tub is half full, add 2 cups (500 ml) of Rose Petal Vinegar.
3. Slip off your clothes and slip into the tub.
4. Relax for 10 to 20 minutes.
5. Rinsing with clear water is optional.

VENUS VINEGAR BATH

This recipe is dedicated to the goddess of love and the goddess present in every woman.

1 cup (250 ml) rose petals
1 cup (250 ml) lemon balm
1 cup (250 ml) calendula blossoms
1 cup (250 ml) comfrey leaves
2 quarts (2 liters) apple cider vinegar

Yield: 4 baths

To make:

1. Collect herbs and flowers fresh, if possible. If using dried, use half the suggested amounts.

2. Spread the herbs and flower petals on paper towels and allow them to wilt overnight.

3. The next day, pour vinegar into a saucepan.

4. Bring to a boil on medium heat.

5. Place the herbs and flower petals in a sterilized widemouthed jar.

6. Pour the vinegar over the petals.

7. Cap the jar with a nonmetal lid and steep for 2 weeks.

8. Strain and bottle in sterilized vinegar bottles.

9. Cork or cap and decorate with stickers, raffia, and ribbons.

To use:

1. Begin drawing a tub of warm water.

2. When the tub is half full, add 2 cups (500 ml) of Venus Vinegar.

3. Slip off your clothes and slip into the tub.

4. Relax for 10 to 20 minutes.

5. Rinsing with clear water is optional.

HERBAL INFUSION BATHS

An herbal infusion is basically a very strong herbal tea. The infusion is created by steeping herbs for 20 minutes up to 4 hours. (See pages 23–24 for instructions on how to brew herbal tea.)

Any herbal tea blend you might drink will also work well in the bath. Don't limit yourself to these recipes; use them as a starting place for developing your own bath blends with your favorite herbs.

COMFREY INFUSION BATH

*C*omfrey is used externally for sprains, strains, and even broken bones. This recipe works best when made fresh, but it will keep 3 days in the refrigerator.

2 tablespoons (30 ml) fresh comfrey (1 tablespoon [15 ml] dried)

2 cups (500 ml) boiling water

Yield: 1 bath treatment

To make:

1. Place the comfrey in a 1-pint (475-ml) jar.
2. Pour boiling water over the comfrey and steep, covered, for 20 minutes to 4 hours.
3. Strain out the herbs, reserving the liquid for the bath.

To use:

1. Add the 2 cups (500 ml) of herbal infusion to a tub half full of warm water.
2. Slip off your clothes and slip into the tub.
3. Relax in the tub for 10 to 20 minutes.
4. Rinse with clear, tepid water.
5. Pat dry.

APHRODITE'S PLEASURE BATH

This recipe is best used freshly made, but it will last 3 days in the refrigerator.

2 tablespoons (30 ml) fresh rose petals (1 tablespoon [15 ml] dried)

2 tablespoons (30 ml) fresh comfrey (1 tablespoon [15 ml] dried)

2 tablespoons (30 ml) fresh elderflowers (1 tablespoon [15 ml] dried)

2 cups (500 ml) boiling water

Yield: 1 treatment

To make:
1. Place the herbs in a 1-pint (475-ml) jar.
2. Pour boiling water over the herbs and steep, covered, for 20 minutes to 4 hours.
3. Strain the liquid for use in the bath.

To use:
1. Add the 2 cups (500 ml) of herbal tea to a tub half full of warm water.
2. Slip off your clothes and slip into the tub.
3. Relax in the tub for 10 to 20 minutes.
4. Rinse with tepid water.
5. Pat dry.

MILK BATHS

Milk baths were a favorite of Cleopatra. The fat of the milk is nourishing to the skin, especially to dry skin. Those with oily skin may choose lower-fat varieties or even nonfat milk powder.

EASY MILK BATH

1. Add 1 quart (1 liter) of milk to a tub half full of warm water.
2. Slip in and relax for 10 to 20 minutes.
3. Rinse with cool water.
4. Pat dry.

COMPRESSES AND POULTICES

Compresses and poultices are techniques for bathing small areas where you may have a breakout, cut, bruise, sprain, or other injury. Using compresses or fomentation is a great way to speed the healing process.

COMFREY COMPRESS FOR SPRAINS AND STRAINS

2 tablespoons (30 ml) fresh herbs (1 tablespoon [15 ml] dried)
2 cups (500 ml) boiling water
Clean cloth, either linen, cotton, or gauze

Yield: 1 treatment

To make:
1. Place the herbs in a clean, 20-ounce (567-g) jar.
2. Pour boiling water over the herbs and steep, covered, for 5 to 20 minutes.
3. Strain the herbs from the infusion and pour remaining liquid into a saucepan.

To use:
1. Reheat the infusion on a low simmer.
2. Remove from heat and put the cloth in the liquid.
3. While still hot, remove the cloth and wring it so it does not drip too much.
4. Place the cloth, as hot as possible, over the affected area. Heat enhances the action of the herbs, so using a hot water bottle to keep the compress warm for 20 minutes is helpful. Be sure to throw the cloth away when you are finished with it.

MAKING A POULTICE FROM A SOCK

Poultices are often used to soothe ankles, wrists, elbows, and feet. An easy way to get all of the healing benefits of the herbs and heat without a lot of fuss and muss is to make a poultice using a cotton sock.

1. Cut the sock above the foot portion.

2. Place 1 cup (250 ml) of dried herbs in a small bowl.

3. Pour ½ cup (125 ml) of boiling water over the herbs.

4. Using a strainer, scoop up the hot herbal material, allow the water to drain, and pour the herbs into the toe area of the sock. The herbs will fill approximately one-third of the sock.

5. Wrap the rest of the sock around the toe portion — poultice — and place it on the sore or sprained elbow, ankle, wrist, or foot.

6. Use the elasticized portion of the sock to secure the poultice in place. Leave the poultice on until it cools.

CHAPTER 20
Herbs for the Feet and Hands
▼▼▼

If you stop for a moment to think about how much your feet and hands do for you each day, you'll appreciate the value of time spent nurturing and caring for these hard-working extremities. I've included recipes to nourish and care for the nails, making them stronger and less brittle, as well as recipes for softening and moisturizing the skin of the feet and hands.

Gardeners often have abused hands. Anyone who works with their hands, from plasterers to masons to artists, will benefit from the formulas in this chapter. They're designed to help counter the drying effects of all the things our hands manage to find their way into.

EQUIPMENT FOR HAND AND FOOT CARE

You are probably familiar with many of the tools of the trade for hand and foot care. All of these items can be purchased at a pharmacy or health and beauty store. I have had a little more

▼▼▼▼
A DIET FOR HEALTHY NAILS

Eating a healthy diet is especially important for healthy nails. Too little protein can make your nails brittle and dull. Deficiencies in vitamins and minerals can also show up in the nails. Be sure to eat those leafy green vegetables and fresh fruits.

Herbal tea can also improve your fingernails over time. Drinking 1 to 3 cups (250 to 750 ml) per day, you should notice improvement in 3 weeks. Yes, iced tea works just as well as hot.

The best herbal teas for healthy nails include borage, chamomile, nettle, oat straw, peppermint, and rose hips.

▲▲▲▲

trouble finding a nail buffer, but it's worth the search, since it helps natural nails glow. The following is a list of the tools you need.

For nail treatments:

- Emery board (not a metal file)
- Nail clippers
- Orange stick
- Finger bowls
- Hand basin (large enough to submerge both hands simultaneously)
- Hand towel
- White fingernail pencil
- Nail buffer

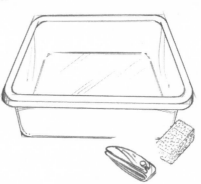

For foot treatments:

- Toenail clippers
- Pumice stone
- Basin

HERBAL NAIL CREAMS AND OILS

Quite a while ago, I met a woman at my workplace who had the most fabulous fingernails. I assumed they must be fake, but found out otherwise when I asked her about them. She told me her secret to long, healthy nails — a small container of an oil mixture that she had purchased commercially and used faithfully every day. Immediately, I went out and purchased the fingernail-polish-size bottle of oil, which cost close to ten dollars. It's quite an ingenious little product; works well, and is all natural. It even helps to dry nail polish.

I didn't think about the price too much at the time, since beauty products can be expensive. But when I got the product home and read the ingredients, I thought, why would ½ ounce (14 g) of this mixture cost nearly ten dollars when I can buy an

8-ounce (227-g) bottle of each ingredient for less than five dollars apiece? The answer is, of course, that the merchant is charging for the cost involved in mixing them together, packaging them in a pretty bottle, advertising, and selling retail. You can avoid paying those high costs by making your own, quite simply. Who knows, maybe you will develop an even better recipe than this one and make your fortune with it!

FABULOUS FINGERNAILS OIL

Nail dryness and brittleness are often the cause of nail breakage — this recipe can help!

1 teaspoon (5 ml) almond oil
1 teaspoon (5 ml) apricot kernel oil
1 teaspoon (5 ml) castor oil
1 teaspoon (5 ml) grapeseed oil
1 teaspoon (5 ml) olive oil
3 drops vitamin E oil
2 drops frankincense essential oil
2 drops benzoin resin

Yield: 2-month supply

To make:
1. Combine all oils and resin in a small amber glass bottle (Boston round) and mix thoroughly by shaking.
2. Keep refrigerated between uses.

To condition nails:
1. Using a cotton swab, apply liberally to the fingernail and cuticle.
2. Massage gently into the fingernail and cuticle.

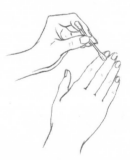

To use as a nail polish dryer:
1. Recycle a nail polish brush by cleaning it with nail polish remover and then soap and water. (You may be able to purchase a single new brush at a health and beauty store.)
2. Apply a thin coat of oil gently over just-applied nail polish, using smooth, even strokes.
3. Allow to air-dry.

HORSETAIL NAIL CREAM

◥◥◥

This cream is especially good for nourishing and protecting the nails. Horsetail, considered a weed, is high in silica, which is found in healthy hair and nails. Make this recipe in the spring, when horsetail is in bloom. Get out your plant identification books and go out and gather it yourself. I think horsetail looks like a miniature (4-inch [10-cm]) Christmas tree. In a pinch, you can use dried horsetail. Benzoin gum resin is great for the nail bed and cuticles, conditioning where you need it most. These make great gifts.

1 cup (250 ml) fresh or ½ cup (125 ml) dried horsetail
1¼ cups (310 ml) olive oil
2 tablespoons (30 ml) beeswax
10 drops vitamin E oil
5 drops benzoin resin
30 ¼-ounce (7-gram) containers with lids

Yield: 30 ¼-ounce (7-gram) containers

To make:
1. Place the fresh horsetail on a towel and allow it to wilt overnight.
2. In a double boiler, steep the horsetail in olive oil over low heat for 3 hours.
3. Grate the beeswax.
4. Strain the plant material out of the oil completely, then pour the oil back into the double boiler. Add the grated beeswax.
5. Heat the mixture until the beeswax melts completely, then remove from heat.
6. Quickly add the vitamin E oil and benzoin gum resin.
7. Pour into dainty ¼-ounce (7-gram) containers or jars and decorate, if desired.

To use:
1. Place your thumb into the container, coating it liberally with nail cream.
2. Systematically massage the cream into each fingernail and cuticle bed.
3. Use twice daily and watch your fingernails improve.

PAPAYA CUTICLE SOAK

This recipe is great for hangnail sufferers. Papaya contains an enzyme that softens and dissolves the undesired cuticle. Regular care of the nails can help to eliminate cuticle problems, even for those who work their hands hard.

2 tablespoons (30 ml) papaya juice
2 tablespoons (30 ml) wheat germ oil
1 teaspoon (5 ml) olive oil

Yield: 1 treatment

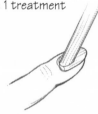

To make:

1. In a blender, combine the juice and wheat germ oil. Run blender on the highest setting for 2 minutes.

To use:

1. Pour juice mixture into a small finger bowl.
2. Measure olive oil into a separate small dish.
3. Soak each hand in the juice mixture for 5 minutes, then rinse with tepid water.
4. Dip an orange stick into the olive oil, then use it to push back the cuticle on each finger.
5. Massage the olive oil into the cuticle.

GELATIN NAIL SOAK

Gelatin is another ingredient that helps build healthy nails and hair. Eating gelatin or taking gelatin supplements improves fingernail strength. External use of gelatin is also helpful.

½ packet gelatin
½ cup (125 ml) boiling water

Yield: 1 treatment

To make:

1. Place gelatin in a small glass bowl and pour boiling water over it. Mix well.
2. Allow gelatin mixture to cool to just warm.

To use:

1. While the mixture is still warm, soak your fingertips in it for 5 minutes.
2. Remove fingertips from bowl and massage the gelatin that remains on your fingers into the nail and nail bed.
3. Rinse with warm water.

HERBAL NAIL COLOR

Do you like the look of nail color but abhor the odor of commercial nail polish? Try henna or alkanet nail color, and buff for a subtle but fashionable look without the aroma.

ALKANET ROOT NAIL OIL

Alkanet root is known for its ability to color oils. It is a great addition to lip gloss and nail color because it has emollient properties as well. Alkanet can be grown in your garden, where you can enjoy the pretty violet flowers before using the root. Ask for seeds at your garden shop. Vary the amount of alkanet — use a little to achieve a blush pink color; use more for darker shades.

3 tablespoons (45 ml) olive oil
½ teaspoon (2 ml) alkanet root
¼ teaspoon (1 ml) beeswax
2 drops vitamin E oil

Yield: Several treatments; good for 1 year if refrigerated

To make:
1. Combine the olive oil and alkanet root in a double boiler.
2. Strain out the alkanet root with a fine mesh strainer, pouring the oil back into the double boiler.
3. Add the beeswax and heat until it melts.
4. Add the vitamin E to the oil, mix, and pour into a small dish or container.

To use:
1. Dip a small brush into the oil and paint your nails, being careful to avoid getting any of the mixture on the surrounding skin.
2. Allow the oil to dry, then reapply.
3. You may want to reapply several times to get a deeper red color.
4. Refrigerate unused portion.

Alkanet

HENNA NAIL PASTE

Henna is not just for the hair — it can also be used to color nails naturally. Experiment with all the different shades to find one that complements your coloring. I love the tawny, earthy tone of brown henna. Orange henna and the black hennas also create interesting shades. Arab women use henna for spiritual protection and to bring prosperity.

1 tablespoon (15 ml) henna
1 tablespoon (15 ml) water
2 drops vitamin E oil

Yield: 1 treatment

To make:
1. Place the henna in a small dish and pour water over it.
2. Add the vitamin E and mix to form a paste.
To use:
1. While the paste is still warm, use a small brush to carefully apply paste to the fingernails only. Wash off any spills on your hands as soon as they occur or you will end up with colorful skin.
2. Allow henna to dry on the nails for at least 20 minutes, or until completely dry.
3. Rinse hands with warm water.
4. Buff nails with nail buffer.

MEHNDI OR HENNA TATTOOS

If you have some leftover henna, try your hand at creating temporary tattoos for kids (or yourself, if that's your thing!). Egyptian and Indian women use henna to paint intricate designs on their hands, a long-standing cultural tradition. Use a toothpick to create fine line drawings. Be sure to let one color of henna dry before applying another color or they will bleed together. Note: The henna will take a few weeks to totally wash off.

HAND-SOFTENING CREAMS

These recipes are especially nice for chapped hands caused by overexposure or by working with drying ingredients. In the winter be sure to wear gloves and drink enough water each day.

HAPPY HANDS HAND CREAM

Everyone loves this cream, but it is especially good for dry skin. Note: The proportions in this recipe are designed for success when combined in a standard kitchen blender; a food processor will not work.

Because of spoilage problems due to rancidity, unused jars of cream must be refrigerated. Package the cream in containers that are opaque or dark to protect them from the destabilizing effects of light. I keep one cream out on my vanity and the rest take up space in my refrigerator.

⅓ cup (80 ml) grape-
    seed oil
⅓ cup (80 ml) olive oil
⅓ cup (80 ml)
    coconut oil
 1 tablespoon (15 ml)
    zinc oxide paste
 1 teaspoon (5 ml)
    cocoa butter
 1 tablespoon (15 ml)
    beeswax
⅓ cup (80 ml) orange
    blossom water
⅓ cup (80 ml) dis-
    tilled water
⅓ cup (80 ml) aloe
    vera gel
20 drops vitamin E oil
 5 drops essential oil
    of orange blossom
 5 drops essential oil
    of frankincense

Yield: 15 1-ounce (25-gram) opaque jars

To make:

1. In a double boiler, melt the grapeseed, olive, and coconut oils; zinc oxide paste; cocoa butter; and beeswax.

2. Once the beeswax is melted, pour the oil mixture into a glass measuring cup, preferably one with a spout.

3. Let cool to room temperature for approximately 1 hour.

4. Set up your 15 clean 1-ounce (25-gram) jars on the edge of your counter for easy pouring.

5. Combine the orange blossom and distilled water, aloe vera gel, and vitamin E and the essential oils in the blender and turn to the highest speed for a minute or two.

6. While the blender is still going, slowly drizzle the cooled oils into the vortex of the waters.

7. Listen to the blender; when it chokes, the water and oil have combined. Turn off the blender.

8. Pour cream into jars and decorate with stickers, ribbon, or labels.

HONEY PASTE

This formula is excellent for softening the most abused hands. It contains ingredients that are emollient and exfoliating at the same time, thus working to remove dry skin while softening the new skin. This recipe can also be used on the feet. It is best applied at bedtime, covered with gloves made of natural fiber, and then left on to work all night.

1 tablespoon (15 ml) almonds
1 tablespoon (15 ml) oatmeal
1 tablespoon (15 ml) zinc oxide paste
1 egg yolk
1 tablespoon (15 ml) honey
1 pair soft kid or cotton gloves

Yield: 1 treatment

To make:

1. In a coffee grinder or spice mill, roughly grind the almonds and the oatmeal, leaving some grit.

2. In a bowl, combine the ground almonds and oatmeal with the zinc oxide paste, egg yolk, and honey, stirring well.

To use:

1. Rub the paste into your hands.

2. Recruit someone to help you put on gloves over your paste-covered hands.

3. Go to sleep for the night, allowing the paste to work its magic. *Note:* You may not want to sleep on your best sheets and bedding if you are concerned about dripping or staining.

4. In the morning, remove the gloves, rinse your hands with cool water, and feel the softness.

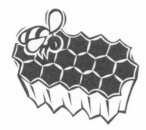

HERBAL PARAFFIN HAND TREATMENTS

This recipe is similar to those you might be treated with in a spa salon. Prepare it in a large, 3-pound (1-kilogram) coffee can so you can dip your entire hand into it, and your elbows, too. If you don't want to make that much, prepare a smaller amount and apply to the hands with a paintbrush. Wax treatments help the skin to absorb moisture, and are especially helpful for dry hands. Frankincense has cell-regenerating properties.

24 ounces (678 g) paraffin wax

4 ounces (113 g) beeswax

1 cup (250 ml) apricot kernel oil

20 drops vitamin E oil

8 drops frankincense essential oil

8 drops lavender essential oil

Yield: 12 hand treatments

To make:

1. In a double boiler, melt the waxes and apricot kernel oil on low heat.

2. Once melted, remove from heat and pour the wax mixture into a clean, large (3-pound [1-kilogram]) coffee can. Be sure the can does not have any sharp edges.

3. Add the vitamin E and essential oils and stir well with a chopstick or spoon.

To use:

1. First apply the Happy Hands Hand Cream (see recipe on page 303) or another hand cream thoroughly and liberally, massaging the cream into your hands.

2. While the wax is still warm but not too hot, dip one hand and then the other into the wax.

3. Allow the wax to air-cool and harden, approximately 20 minutes.

4. Gently peel off the paraffin and discard. Note: You can store the leftover wax right in the coffee can by placing the lid on it, but be sure to use it within 1 year. To use again, reheat and melt in a water bath. You may choose to add more essential oil and vitamin E, as they will dissipate with reheating.

HERBAL FOOTBATHS AND SOAKS

Many herbs are delightful to use in a footbath, and footbaths are delightful because you enjoy an aromatherapy session at the same time. Any herbs that you might use for external use or drink as tea are generally good for baths. The herbs are prepared the same way as herbal infusions (see page 292). Footbaths are simple to prepare, and your feet definitely deserve some pampering.

CAUTION

The treatments presented in this chapter are beneficial for addressing a wide range of health concerns. However, you should consult your doctor before engaging in the treatments, especially if you have varicose veins or circulation or heart problems.

HERBAL FOOTBATH

2 cups (500 ml) fresh herbs of your choice (1 cup [250 ml] dried)
Boiling water

Yield: 1 treatment

To make:

1. Select desired herb or herb combination (see box) and place in a 1-quart (1-liter) jar.

2. Pour boiling water over the herbs, cover tightly, and allow to steep for 20 minutes.

To use:

1. Strain the liquid from the herbs (called an herbal infusion) into a foot basin.

2. Add warm water to achieve the level and temperature desired. Use care in your choice of temperature: 100° to 110°F is best.

3. Submerge your feet and relax for 10 minutes.

4. Enlist a friend to rub your feet while they are in the water and to pat them dry when finished, or you can do this for yourself.

OLIVE OIL SOFTENING SOAK

Also great for the fingernails, this recipe contains olive oil infused with sage, horsetail, and red clover. It is helpful for brittle nails and for calluses. I like to make enough for the feet and use the rest on my hands and fingertips, but you can make a smaller batch just for your hands. For sanitary purposes, make a fresh batch for each individual.

3 ounces (85 g) fresh horsetail
3 ounces (85 g) fresh red clover
3 ounces (85 g) fresh sage
2 cups (500 ml) olive oil
5 drops vitamin E oil
5 drops vanilla essential oil
1 16-ounce (454-gram) amber-colored bottle (Boston round) or two 8-ounce (227-gram) bottles

Yield: 2 cups (500 ml)

To make:

1. Gather the fresh herbs and lay them on a paper towel to wilt overnight. (This allows for any dew or water on the plant material to evaporate, thereby protecting your oil from contamination.)
2. The next day, combine the oil and wilted herbs in a double boiler.
3. Simmer on low for 4 hours.
4. Strain the plant material, reserving the oil.
5. Add the vitamin E oil and essential oil to this mixture.
6. Pour into the amber bottle(s).

To use:

1. Pour 1 cup of oil into a warm-water footbath.
2. Submerse both feet and relax for 10 minutes.
3. Enlist a friend to rub your feet while they are in the water and to pat them dry when finished, or you can do this part yourself.

HERBS FOR TIRED FEET

- Agrimony
- Alder
- Burdock
- Comfrey
- Elderberry
- Lavender
- Mugwort
- Pine
- Red clover
- Rosemary
- Sage

HOT AND COLD FOOTBATH

Hot and cold stimulation is great for the entire body and especially help-ful to the feet. I like using it after ice skating and skiing. You will be amazed at how good this simple procedure feels. If you suffer from cir-culation or other health problems, be sure to check with your doctor before doing this treatment.

In place of the hot water in this recipe, you can use the herbal infu-sion or olive oil soak (see pages 306–307) for the hot bath and thus receive the benefit of the herbs and oils.

2 foot basins
Hot water to fill basin
⅔ full
Cold water to fill basin
⅔ full

Yield: 1 treatment

To make:
1. Heat hot-water bath to 100° to 110°F.
2. Make cold-water bath 50°F.
To use:
1. Starting with the basin of hot water, submerse your feet for 5 minutes.
2. Remove your feet from the hot water and place them in the cold-water basin for 2 minutes.
3. Go back to the hot and repeat as desired, being sure to finish with the cold.
4. Pat dry.

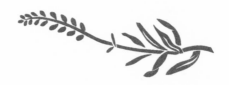

HERBAL FOOT SCRUBS

Any number of ingredients can be used for making foot scrubs. The recipes for facial scrubs in chapter 16 are almost as effective for the feet as they are for the face. You may have heard of the benefits of walking in sand with bare feet: Sand can also be used as an ingredient in foot scrubs. Avocado pit meal and avocado skins are great, too, and you get to make use of parts you would just be throwing out otherwise.

While you might use facial recipes on your feet, I don't recommend using foot scrub recipes on the delicate skin on your face and body. They're best for the tougher skin of the feet, elbows, and knees.

A WALK ON THE BEACH

1 cup (250 ml) sand (coarseness of your choice)

1 tablespoon (15 ml) sea salt

1 tablespoon (15 ml) powdered dulse

1 tablespoon (15 ml) powdered kelp

1 cup (250 ml) olive oil

2 foot basins

Yield: 2 treatments

To make:

1. Place the sand, salt, and seaweeds in a bowl.

2. Pour the olive oil over the mixture, mixing well.

To use:

1. Place your feet in a foot basin. Massage the sand mixture into both feet, giving special care to your heels.

2. Move feet to second basin and rinse your feet with cool water.

3. Repeat the treatment, and rinse again in cool water.

4. Pat dry.

AVOCADO SKIN SOFTENER

Avocados help soften and remove calluses. Each part of the avocado has a different use. The ground pit makes a wonderful emollient scrub, the pulp is a rich moisturizer that is especially good for dry skin, and the skin of the fruit contains a potent cosmetic oil. Application of this formula will dissolve dead skin and make your feet feel satiny smooth.

1 avocado pit
½ avocado
¼ cup (60 ml) cornmeal
1 tablespoon (15 ml) sea salt

Yield: 1 treatment

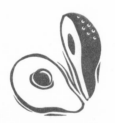

To make:

1. Dry out the avocado pit for a few days, then break into several pieces.

2. In a spice mill or coffee grinder, grind the pit to make gritty avocado pit meal.

3. Reserving its skin, mash the ½ avocado with the cornmeal, ¼ cup (50 ml) avocado pit meal, and sea salt.

To use:

1. In a foot basin, gently massage the mixture into your feet in a circular motion, starting with the toes.

2. Massage the scrub into the ball of each foot working into and around all the little bones there.

3. Massage and stroke the arches.

4. With a bit more pressure, work on the heels and the outside of the foot.

5. Massage the ankles and the tops of the feet.

6. Rinse with tepid water.

7. With the inner (sticky) side of the avocado skin, rub the heel and any other callused areas including your knees, elbows, and hands. Do not rinse off. Massage the oil into the skin with your hands in gentle, circular motions.

8. At first your skin may seem green, but keep massaging. Soon you'll feel the abrasive effects, then the moisturizing effects.

PUMICE FOOT EXFOLIATION

You can purchase pumice stones at any pharmacy. I like to use mine while bathing, but a pumice stone scrub can also be combined with any of the preceding foot treatments. A pumice stone treatment accompanied by a reflexology rub makes a much appreciated "hands-on" gift for a friend or loved one.

Pumice stone
Soap
Water

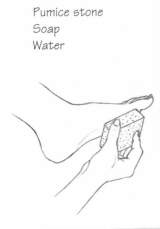

To use:

1. Soften your feet by soaking them in water or an herb bath for a few minutes.

2. Wash the feet thoroughly.

3. In a circular motion, rub the pumice stone around all parts of the feet.

4. Rinse with tepid water.

5. Pat dry.

REFLEXOLOGY FOOT MASSAGE

Reflexology is a method for activating the healing powers of the body through massage techniques applied to the feet (or hands). More than just a simple foot rub (not to diminish the value of that) however, reflexology is a systematic approach to the feet, taking into account any health problems. It is based on the principle that there are energy zones (referred to as meridians by the acupuncturist or Chinese healer) that run through the body and the feet. These areas reflect or "reflex" and correspond to all the organs, glands, and other parts of the whole body. Similar to the concept of a hologram, which always contains the whole, by working on the corresponding spots on the feet or the hands, you can affect the whole body.

For a more in-depth appreciation of reflexology, consult your bookstore or library. There are also training programs specifically set up to teach and certify individuals in the art and science of reflexology. Many manicurists and pedicurists are familiar with the techniques; you may want to indulge in a professional treatment with one of them and consult about how to practice at home.

DEODORIZING AND CURATIVE FOOT TREATMENTS

Our feet do much for us each day and, sadly, they are often the most neglected part of our bodies. Be sure to pamper your feet, and treat them to footbaths, foot rubs, and invigorating foot powders every now and then.

HERBAL FOOT POWDER

This powder is easy to make, at a fraction of the cost of commercial products, and contains only all-natural ingredients — how can you lose? The elderberry helps reduce fatigue. Some of the old herbals recommend putting elder flowers or leaves in your shoes. Lovage is one of my favorite aromatics and is a natural deodorant. Note: This powder may also be used as a body powder (see recipe on page 319).

½ cup (125 ml) dried elder flowers or leaves

½ cup (125 ml) dried lovage

1 cup (250 ml) white clay

2 cups (500 ml) cornstarch

8 drops peppermint essential oil

Powder cylinders or a recycled powder puff and container

Yield: 4 cups (1 liter)

To make:

1. In a spice mill or coffee grinder, grind the elder flowers and then the lovage to a fine powder.

2. In a large bowl, combine all dry ingredients, mixing with a wire whisk.

3. Scent with essential oil, and again mix with the wire whisk.

4. Allow mixture to sit overnight, covered with a towel, to fix the scent.

5. In the morning, mix again with a wire whisk.

6. Package in powder cylinders.

To use:

1. Sprinkle powder in your shoes before putting them on in the morning.

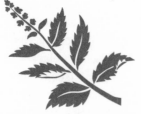

CORN CURE

1 garlic clove for each
corn

Yield: 1 treatment

To make:
1. Roast garlic cloves.
To use:
1. While hot, apply a whole garlic clove directly to a corn.
2. Place a bandage over each corn and garlic clove.
3. Repeat application for 3 to 4 days, until corns loosen and fall off. (You'll keep vampires away at the same time!)

ATHLETE'S FOOT CURE

You won't find this cure in any luxury spas, but it won't cost you a dime and is highly effective. Urine, or urea, is slightly acidic and is an ingredient in many beauty products, valued for its healing properties and the fact that it is closer to the natural pH of the skin. Uncontaminated urine is highly sanitary, pure, and antiseptic. It was used on battlefields for surgery and works particularly well on jellyfish stings. Some ancient cultures bathed in urine as a beauty ritual. Eastern cultures use urine for beauty and for healing. Also works well on warts, including plantar's warts.

1 cup (250 ml) urine
from the person
being treated
1 gallon (4 liters)
warm water

Yield: 1 treatment

To make:
1. In a foot basin, combine the urine and warm water.
To use:
1. Soak feet for 20 minutes.
2. Rinse with cool water.
Variation: If you cannot bring yourself to use urine, substitute ½ cup lemon juice or apple cider vinegar. This combination will require more frequent treatments, but it is effective because of the acidity. Nonalkaline soap is also helpful, as is a black walnut hull herbal infusion footbath (see recipe on page 306 and substitute black walnut hulls, which have antifungal properties, for the herbs).

CHAPTER 21

Herbal Hygiene

▼▼▼▼▼

Throughout the centuries, people in various cultures have used herbal products to stay fresh and clean. Herbal teas have traditionally been used for internal cleansing. Herbal mouthwashes and gargles keep breath fresh and can also help with oral hygiene. Herbal tooth powders are easy to make and leave the teeth feeling smooth. A variety of aromatic herbs lend themselves to scenting body powders. Herbal underarm deodorant can keep you feeling fresh.

HERBAL TEAS

Herbal beverages can help keep the body fresh and clean. Drinking eight glasses of water daily also helps keep the body fresh by helping it excrete toxins.

BODY-FRESHENING TEA

▼▼▼▼▼

Almost any herbal tea will help freshen your body, but the ones listed here are notable for their body odor–defying qualities. Increase the amount of herbs and water proportionally to brew as many cups as you desire. It is best to make it fresh daily, but it can be refrigerated for two days.

8 ounces (227 g) water
1 tablespoon (15 ml) of one of the following fresh herbs (1 teaspoon [5 ml] dried):
  Lovage
  Sagebrush
  Peppermint
  Cleavers
  Thyme

Yield: 1 cup

To make:
1. Bring the water to a boil.
2. Place the herbs in a jar and pour the boiling water over them; cover.
3. Steep flowers briefly for 5 minutes; steep leafy material for 20 minutes. Strain out herbs and reserve liquid.
To use:
1. Drink 3 cups per day for best results.

314

HERBAL MOUTHWASH AND GARGLE

Herbal mouthwash and gargle is yet another product that is easy to make and use, and it doesn't have any of the chemicals common in many commercial products. Do remember that serious breath problems are often the result of poor digestion. Consult with your physician if in doubt.

CINNAMON SPICE MOUTHWASH

1 tablespoon (15 ml) cinnamon chips

1 tablespoon (15 ml) whole cloves

1 teaspoon (5 ml) anise seed

1 teaspoon (5 ml) ground nutmeg

1 cup (250 ml) vodka

Yield: 16 treatments

To make:

1. Place all the spices in a clean glass jar.

2. Pour the vodka over the spices, cap, and shake daily for the next 2 weeks.

3. Strain and pour into a dark amber bottle.

To use:

1. This mouthwash is concentrated. Use 1 tablespoon mouthwash dissolved in 1 cup (250 ml) water.

2. Gargle as usual.

3. Rinse with clear, cool water.

DIET FOR A FRESH-SMELLING BODY

Diet is a major contributor to body odor, as are hormonal fluctuations. A vegetarian diet or one high in fruits and vegetables reduces body odor because chlorophyll, a substance naturally found in green plants, helps control the bacteria that cause body odor. Parsley, beet greens, and lovage have a cleansing effect on both the breath and body odors.

MINTY MOUTHWASH

½ cup (125 ml)
   spearmint
½ cup (125 ml)
   peppermint
1 cup (250 ml) white
   wine

Yield: 16 treatments

To make:

1. Place the herbs in a clean glass jar.

2. Pour the white wine over the herbs, cap, and shake daily for the next 2 weeks.

3. Strain and pour into a dark amber bottle.

To use:

1. This mouthwash is concentrated. Use 1 tablespoon mouthwash dissolved in 1 cup (250 ml) water.

2. Gargle as usual.

3. Rinse with clear, cool water.

LAVENDER-PEPPERMINT MOUTH RINSE

*S*earching for a nonalcoholic product? Look no further. Since there is no alcohol to preserve this recipe, it must be made fresh each time.

1 tablespoon (15 ml)
   fresh lavender (1 tea-
   spoon [5 ml] dried)
1 tablespoon (15 ml)
   peppermint (1 tea-
   spoon [5 ml] dried)
1 cup (250 ml) water

Yield: 1 treatment

To make:

1. Bring the water to a boil.

2. Add the herbs to a clean glass jar.

3. Pour the boiling water over the herbs and let steep for 30 minutes.

4. Strain.

To use:

1. Gargle with the strong herbal tea.

BREATH-FRESHENING HERBS

Cloves, fennel seed, parsley, peppermint, spearmint, watercress, and wintergreen are useful to freshen the breath.

I like to chew on fresh wintergreen, parsley, or the mints. The spices, fennel, and cloves can be used dried; simply chew on them. Use these herbs and spices in place of breath mints and avoid the added sugar and artificial sweeteners.

Factors that may contribute to chronic breath odor are inadequate diet and stomach and other health problems. Bad breath should be checked by a health-care provider if it persists.

HERBAL TOOTH CARE

Tooth powders are fun and easy to make. The baking soda produces a naturally fresh, clean feeling in the mouth, while affecting its pH and making it less acidic.

HERBAL TOOTH POWDER

Myrrh powder is added to this recipe to help prevent periodontal disease. Baking soda, an ingredient in many commercial products, lessens the mouth's acidity. Raspberry leaf is good for the gums and mildly astringent. Tea tree oil is effective against gingivitis and plaque buildup; the yellow dock is cleansing.

½ cup (125 ml) baking soda

½ cup (125 ml) white clay powder

1 teaspoon (5 ml) dried raspberry leaf

1 teaspoon (5 ml) dried yellow dock root

1 teaspoon (5 ml) myrrh powder

1 teaspoon (5 ml) flavoring herbs of your choice (fennel, peppermint, spearmint, wintergreen)

5 drops essential oil of tea tree

Yield: about 1 cup (250 ml)

To make:

1. Pour the baking soda and white clay powder into a medium-size mixing bowl.

2. In a spice mill or coffee grinder, grind the dried herbs into a powder.

3. Add all the dry ingredients, including the myrrh powder, to the baking soda–clay mixture.

4. Mix well with a wire whisk.

5. Add the tea tree oil, again mixing well.

6. Place a clean hand towel over the bowl, covering it completely.

7. Let sit overnight.

8. The next morning, mix well again with the wire whisk.

9. Package in an opaque widemouthed jar. It will last indefinitely if you keep moisture out of the package.

To use:

1. Wet your toothbrush, then sprinkle a small quantity of powder onto your brush.

2. Brush thoroughly and gently in an up-and-down motion.

3. Brush the tongue, too.

4. Rinse, and feel the freshness of your mouth.

STRAWBERRY TEETH WHITENER

This recipe leaves the teeth clean and shiny. Strawberries have been used through the centuries for tooth whitening.

3–6 ripe strawberries
2 teaspoons (10 ml) baking soda
1 teaspoon (5 ml) cream of tartar
1 cup water

Yield: 1 treatment

To make:

1. In a blender, purée the berries.

2. Pour the fruit into a small dish.

To use:

1. With your toothbrush or a cosmetic brush, paint a paste of the berries onto your teeth. Let sit on teeth for 5 minutes.

2. Add 1 teaspoon of the baking soda and cream of tartar to the cup of water.

3. Swish the soda water around in your mouth.

4. Brush your teeth with the remaining baking soda.

5. Rinse with cool, clear water.

HERBAL BODY POWDER AND DEODORANTS

I don't recommend using antiperspirant; perspiration is a natural, and necessary, process in a healthy body. Natural deodorants like the following do not block the skin or clog the pores; they do alter the scent of perspiration and affect the bacteria that cause body odor.

HERBAL BODY POWDER

This powder is easy to make and at a fraction of the cost of commercial products. With only natural ingredients, how can you go wrong? Use it in place of deodorant or antiperspirant. It is also effective at preventing the chafing between the thighs that you may experience when bicycle riding or in hot, humid weather.

1 cup (250 ml) white clay

2 cups (500 ml) cornstarch

¼ cup (60 ml) powdered herb of your choice. (Lavender and rose are nice, but any aromatic will work.)

8 drops essential oil

Yield: Approximately 3 cups

To make:

1. Combine all dry ingredients in a large bowl, mixing with a wire whisk.

2. Scent with essential oil and cover with a towel. Allow mix to sit overnight.

3. Remix with the wire whisk, then package in powder cylinders.

GIFT IDEA

Decorate a powder cylinder with floral stickers or recycle a fluffy powder puff and pretty container. This makes a special gift for someone who is on her feet a lot.

LEMON RIND DEODORANT

This is a simple, natural way to stay fresh smelling and feeling.

Rind of 1 lemon

Yield: 1 treatment

To use:
Rub the fleshy side of the lemon rind under your armpits and allow to dry.

THYME AND ORANGE PEEL DEODORANT

More zesty than the Lemon Rind Deodorant, this is also a wonderful way to stay fresh.

¼ cup (60 ml) fresh thyme
Zest of 1 orange
½ cup (125 ml) apple cider vinegar

Yield: 4 ounces (100 g)

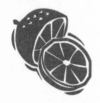

To make:
1. Place the fresh thyme and the orange zest in a jar.
2. Pour the apple cider vinegar over the herbs and cover with a nonmetal lid.
3. Steep the mix for 2 weeks, shaking daily.
To use:
1. Pour 1 tablespoon (15 ml) of the vinegar over two cotton balls.
2. Rub the soaked cotton balls under each arm.

HERBS WITH DEODORIZING PROPERTIES

- ◆ Lemon juice
- ◆ Lovage
- ◆ Orange peel
- ◆ Orrisroot
- ◆ Patchouli
- ◆ Sagebrush
- ◆ Thyme
- ◆ Witch hazel

BAY RUM AFTERSHAVE

Next time you're in California, you have to make this tonic for the man in your life. But don't let him keep it all to himself; it is also a nice toner for women who like spicy scents. This recipe was inspired by the bay rum products offered in many mail-order catalogs.

2 cups (500 ml) fresh bay leaves

1 tablespoon (15 ml) dried, whole cloves

1 teaspoon (5 ml) ground ginger

1 teaspoon (5 ml) allspice

1 teaspoon (5 ml) fennel

2 cups (500 ml) rum

Yield: 2 cups (500 ml)

To make:

1. Fill a widemouthed jar with bay leaves, cloves, ginger, allspice, and fennel.

2. Cover the herbs with rum.

3. Let sit for 4 weeks in a warm place, shaking occasionally.

4. Strain out the herbs and rebottle the herbal liquid.

To use:

1. Dilute with orange blossom floral water (see box on page 255 for proportions).

2. Men should pour approximately 2 tablespoons in their hands, then splash on the face after shaving. Women, you'll feel refreshed splashing some on after washing up.

BLEMISH LINIMENT

Use this ointment on boils, acne, infected wounds, cuts, poison oak, and poison ivy. This recipe is my variation of Jethro Kloss' liniment (see *Back to Eden* for the original).

1 tablespoon (15 ml) dried goldenseal powder

2 tablespoons (30 ml) dried echinacea powder

2 tablespoons (30 ml) dried myrrh powder

2 teaspoons (10 ml) dried cayenne powder

2 cups (500 ml) 100-proof vodka

2 cups (500 ml) distilled water

Yield: 4 cups

To make:

1. Place herbs in a jar and cover with vodka.

2. Shake daily for 4 weeks.

3. Strain and rebottle the liquid, using 1 part liquid to 1 part distilled water.

To use:

1. Dab liniment onto a cotton ball.

2. Lightly rub on affected areas. If it is too harsh, dilute 1:2 instead (1 part liniment to 2 parts distilled water).

CHAPTER 22
Putting It All Together

～～～

It is easy enough to use the recipes in this book on an occasional basis — trying a recipe here and there as you get a chance or as a particular need or desire arises. That's great, but I encourage you to incorporate some of the treatments into your daily self-care routine. You will achieve the greatest benefit to your body if you give yourself these treatments on a regular basis. Following are suggestions for treatment combinations that you could use to develop an ongoing nurturing program.

ESTABLISH A NEW TRADITION

When I was a child, my mother had her card parties. Why not start a tradition of nurturing parties? Maybe you already attend a women's group or a men's group: A few of the treatments could be the focus for a program or even an ongoing focus. Garden clubs that want a creative way to use their harvest can institute programs when herbs and flowers are bountiful.

Schedule Regular Appointments for Yourself

The most important part of any beauty ritual is making the time for it. It is easy for women to put themselves last, scheduling their lives around others. To really be of service to those in your life, you must take time for yourself. It demonstrates to your children the importance of spending time enhancing self-esteem. So get out your calendar. Schedule some treatments, and keep your appointments. You will feel better, and your family will benefit from your greater feelings of fulfillment.

A Chance to Share with Others

Many of the treatment combinations suggested in the following section are similar to those you might find at a resort or day spa. Take this opportunity to share time with your partner or another loved one so you can really enjoy yourself. These treatment combinations make a great gift for a special occasion, such as a birthday, anniversary, or job promotion.

Herbal home spa treatments also offer a nice chance to share an activity with your children, especially daughters. Children love to make some of the easier recipes (e.g., lip balm, soap balls, henna tattoos, or nail color) that they can use themselves and give to their friends as gifts. Children can also learn to give and receive nurturing treatments. A massage is a great chance for you to nurture each other and share the loving touch.

SUGGESTED TREATMENT ROUTINES

You probably already have daily morning and evening cleansing routines. You may be surprised at how little effort it takes to substitute nourishing herbal body treatments for your more conventional ones, and how much better they will make you feel about yourself and your body.

Daily Treatments

In the morning:

- ◆ Use an all-over skin exfoliation technique such as Roman Skin Brushing, Ayate Fiber Rub, Loofah Scrub, or Garshan Silk Mitt Treatment.
- ◆ Cleanse your face using an herbal cleansing milk or gel.
- ◆ Tone skin using floral water or herbal astringent.
- ◆ Apply Violet Eye Cream.
- ◆ Apply nail oil or cream.
- ◆ Massage in a facial cream with sun protection.

In the evening:

- ◆ Use an all-over skin exfoliation technique such as Roman Skin Brushing, Ayate Fiber Rub, Loofah Scrub, or Garshan Silk Mitt Treatment.
- ◆ Cleanse face with avena cleansing grains.
- ◆ Tone skin using floral water or an herbal astringent.

Weekly Treatments

- ◆ Herbal facial steam or Papaya Enzyme Treatment
- ◆ Oxygen Facial or Peel-off Mask
- ◆ Herbal body scrub
- ◆ Herbal bath treatment
- ◆ Scalp treatment
- ◆ Herbal hair rinse

DON'T MOISTURIZE AT NIGHT

Contrary to many skin-care programs, I do not recommend using a moisturizer or night cream on your skin before bed. My experience is that a natural detoxification occurs at night. This process brings the natural oils of the face to the surface, allowing the skin to circulate, breath, and naturally moisturize itself. The use of creams at night blocks these processes.

Monthly Treatments

◆ Herbal foot scrub and bath
◆ Herbal body wrap
◆ Infused oil massage

PLANNING A DAY OF BEAUTY IN YOUR HERBAL HOME SPA

Once you've got your home spa up and running and you've tried some of the treatments, make an appointment for yourself to enjoy a day of beauty there. For best results, prepare as much as you can a day in advance, so you can just sit back and enjoy the treatment. It is also nice to make a special light lunch and have some brewed herbal tea ready so you can enjoy yourself without any work on this relaxing day. Do the treatments in the order suggested here.

HERBAL HOME SPA TREATMENT PROGRAMS

Full-Day Program One	Full-Day Program Two	Half-Day Program
Roman Dry Brushing	Flower Essence Scalp Massage	Ayate Fiber Rub
Oatmeal Almond Body Scrub	Violet Eye Cream	Seaweed Body Wrap
Rose Petal Vinegar Bath	Herbal Facial Steam	Papaya Enzyme Facial Treatment
Cucumber Eye Pack	Peel-off Mask	Deep Pore Treatment
Oxygen Facial	Floral Water	Queen of Hungary Water
Paraffin Hand and Foot Treatment	Garshan Silk Mitt Treatment	Lip Balm
Creamy Lotion Full-body Massage	Cellulite Body Wrap	Lavender Blue Face Moisturizer
	Hot and Cold Stimulation	
	Rose Pink Face Moisturizer	

APPENDIX:
A Guide to Ingredients

This chapter is a descriptive journey through my "green world." I use all of the natural ingredients that follow in the personal care products I make for myself and my friends, family, and clients. By adopting at least a few of these ingredients into your skin care repertoire, you will be educating yourself about what you put in and on your body. Only you can take control of your skin's health!

BASE OILS

Base oils are derived from nuts, seeds, vegetables, and fruits. They have mild therapeutic properties, but as the name implies, they are most often used as a base or carrier oil to which essential oils and herbs are added when making oils, lotions, or creams.

The best oils to purchase for skin care purposes are cold- or expeller-pressed, as they are not extracted at extremely high temperatures and/or with a chemical solvent. (Exposure to high temperatures and chemical solvents can destroy natural flavors, aromas, antioxidant properties, and beneficial trace minerals and vitamins.) Cold-pressed oils are processed at a relatively low temperature (150–250°F, or 65–120°C). Expeller-pressed oils have been mechanically pressed from the nut, seed, fruit, or vegetable from which it is derived. Cold- and expeller-pressed oils, by the way, are also highly recommended for use in cooking and salad dressings, as they have a better flavor and higher nutritional value than conventionally processed oils.

Base oils, with the exception of avocado, hazelnut, jojoba, and extra-virgin olive, tend to become rancid if stored at room temperature for more than 4 to 6 months; they should be refrigerated. The oils described below should have only a trace of fragrance, if any at all. If the oil has a strong or "off" smell (with the exception of olive oil), then it's probably old. Purchase base oils through reputable mail-order suppliers (see Resources) or better health food stores with a high inventory turnover. Don't hesitate to return the product if it is bad.

ALMOND OIL
Description: A clear to very pale yellow oil pressed from sweet almond seeds (kernels). Full of vitamins and minerals. Reasonably priced and widely available.
Uses: From massage oils to lotions, creams to masks, almond oil is good for all skin types, especially dry, inflamed, or itchy skin. A first-rate, all-purpose oil.

AVOCADO OIL
Description: A clear, medium to dark green oil derived from the fatty fruit pulp. Rich in protein, vitamins, and fatty acids. A very stable oil with a long shelf life. Moderately priced and sometimes difficult to find.
Uses: Especially good blended with other base oils and used as an after-bath body or facial oil — use 1 part avocado oil to 10 parts other base oils. The perfect, nourishing oil for dull, lifeless, dry, and devitalized skin; eczema; and psoriasis.

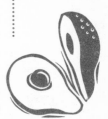

BORAGE SEED OIL
Description: A pale yellow oil pressed from the seeds. Very rich in beneficial GLA (gamma linolenic acid), vitamins, and minerals. Expensive, but worth it.
Uses: Taken internally, borage seed oil lessens PMS symptoms and helps to lubricate joints and skin. When blended with avocado, jojoba, hazelnut, or almond oil, it is used externally to treat eczema, psoriasis, and signs of premature aging. Dilute with other base oils using a 1 to 10 ratio.

CASTOR OIL
Description: A very thick, clear to slightly yellow oil processed from the seeds of an annual shrub. Extremely moisturizing. Inexpensive and easy to find.
Uses: I like it for the staying power and shine it provides to my lip balm and gloss recipes. Particularly good for softening rough, dry heels, knees, elbows, and patches of eczema and psoriasis.

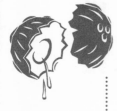

COCONUT PALM OIL

Description: Expressed from coconut meat, this white semisolid fat melts at room temperature. Widely available and inexpensive.

Uses: Excellent as a massage or bath oil or when used in lotions and creams. A mild, gentle oil, good for sensitive and infant skin.

HAZELNUT OIL

Description: A clear, pale yellow oil derived from the pressed kernel, hazelnut oil has a mild, nutty fragrance. High in vitamin E and fatty acids. It has a light, penetrating quality that makes it good for all skin types. Usually only available through mail-order suppliers, moderately priced.

Uses: One of the best base oils used in face creams and lotions because of its lightness and stability (it is not prone to rancidity). Especially good for aging skin.

JOJOBA OIL

Description: Actually a liquid plant wax, this clear, yellow oil is pressed from the seeds. The thick oil closely resembles human sebum in consistency. Will not become rancid; hardens in cold weather. Expensive, but relatively easy to find.

Uses: Good for inflamed skin, eczema, psoriasis, rough or dry skin, and acne. Penetrates easily and is very compatible with human skin.

OLIVE OIL

Description: A clear green oil with a strong olive fragrance taken from the first pressing of ripe olives. High in vitamin E. Moderately priced, widely available. Be sure to choose the extra-virgin variety.

Uses: Though a very high-quality cosmetic oil, I rarely use it, except when combining with salt to make body scrubs or salves, because of its overpowering fragrance and color.

ROSEHIP SEED OIL

Description: Clear, reddish in color, derived from the seeds of the ripened fruit of *Rosa rubiginosa* (commonly known as Rosa Mosqueta). Extremely high in essential fatty acids. Expensive and usually only available from better health food stores or mail-order suppliers.

Uses: Used with much success in treatments for skin damage that has resulted in premature aging, dehydration, wrinkles, or scars. Highly recommended for mature, dry, and sun-damaged skin.

Contraindication: Should not be used on skin that is oily or acneic.

SESAME OIL

Description: Derived from the pressed seeds, this clear, golden oil is rich in vitamins A and E and protein. It's a very stable base oil, meaning that it has a long shelf life.

Uses: Used in sunscreens, salves, and lotions. Superb as a body oil for normal-to-dry skin.

Note: Do not use the toasted varieties of sesame oil in your skin care products.

SOYBEAN OIL

Description: A clear, yellow, highly refined, widely available, inexpensive oil. Commonly found in grocery stores under the label of "vegetable oil." Check the ingredients panel and it should read "100 percent soybean oil."

Uses: A terrific massage oil. Penetrates readily with no greasy residue. Not my number one choice, though, because of the chemical residues found in most brands as a result of processing, but can be used in a pinch. Try to find an organically produced soybean oil.

FRUITS

The following is a list of fruits to use in natural skin care recipes. These fruits contain fruit acids, also called alpha-hydroxy acids (AHAs) or beta-hydroxy agents (BHAs), that are extremely good for the skin when applied externally. AHAs dissolve the bond that holds dead skin cells together and increases hydration while BHAs naturally dissolve dry, flaky surface skin and stimulate cell renewal. All skin types from oily to very dry can benefit from these remarkably effective and inexpensive fruit acids.

When purchasing, try to find organically grown fruit. *Note:* For maximum skin rejuvenation, all fruits should be used in their raw state.

APPLE (AHA)

Parts Used: Pulp, freshly pressed juice

Cosmetic Properties and Uses: Contains malic acid. Acts as a mild astringent. Soothing for sensitive and acneic skin. Mixed with white cosmetic clay, makes a gentle, exfoliating mask.

BANANA (AHA)

Parts Used: Pulp

Cosmetic Properties and Uses: Nourishing and moisturizing. Extremely gentle. Recommended for normal and dry skin. Can be used straight as a mask or blended with white cosmetic clay for added exfoliation and tightening.

BLACKBERRY AND RASPBERRY (AHA)

Parts Used: Freshly pressed, strained juice

Cosmetic Properties and Uses: Contains lactic acid. Can be applied with a cotton ball directly to all but the most sensitive or sunburned skin as an exfoliating tonic and then rinsed off. Moderately astringent.

CITRUS FRUITS — GRAPEFRUIT, LEMON, LIME, ORANGE, TANGERINE (AHA)

Parts Used: Freshly pressed juice, rind (zest)

Cosmetic Properties and Uses: Contains citric acid. Astringent and fragrant. Good for oily and normal skin. Juice and zest can be added to toners, spritzers, masks, and lotions.

Contraindication: Do not use on sensitive or inflamed skin.

GRAPE (AHA)

Parts Used: Freshly pressed juice

Cosmetic Properties and Uses: Contains tartaric acid. Apply juice to face with cotton ball to help improve skin texture, rinse. Safe for all skin types.

PAPAYA (BHA)

Parts Used: Pulp

Cosmetic Properties and Uses: Contains the enzyme papain. Applied as a wet mask, helps even out skin tone and soften skin. Especially useful for a fading tan or dry, flaky skin.

Contraindication: May be irritating to sensitive, sunburned, or inflamed skin.

PINEAPPLE (BHA)
Parts Used: Freshly pressed juice
Cosmetic Properties and Uses: Contains the enzyme bromelain. Will dissolve dead, dry skin cells resulting in smoother skin.
Contraindication: May be irritating to sensitive, sunburned, or inflamed skin.

STRAWBERRY (AHA)
Parts Used: Pulp
Cosmetic Properties and Uses: Acts as a gentle astringent. Safe for all skin types. Pulp may be thickened with white cosmetic clay and applied as an exfoliating mask.

GRAINS, NUTS, AND SEEDS

I always have a generous supply of the following four "skin foods" in my kitchen. They are staples for the kitchen cosmetologist. All ingredients should be organically grown, if possible, and used in raw form. To ensure freshness, nuts and seeds should be kept in the freezer. Oatmeal can be stored in a cool, dry cabinet.

ALMOND
Forms Used: Ground almonds (almond meal)
Cosmetic Properties and Uses: High in skin-loving nutrients and fat. Used as a facial and body scrub base to gently exfoliate rough, dry skin.

FLAXSEED
Forms Used: Ground seeds (flaxseed meal) or cracked seeds
Cosmetic Properties and Uses: When water is added to the whole, cracked seeds or meal, the resulting emollient gel can be strained and massaged into the skin to soothe, nourish, and help heal minor irritations, acne, and sunburn.

OATMEAL

Forms Used: Ground oatmeal

Cosmetic Properties and Uses: Added to bath water, oatmeal relieves itchy, rashy skin and allergic reactions from poison ivy, oak, and sumac or insect bites. Ground oatmeal can also be used as a mask base for all skin types and as a gentle facial scrub for sensitive or couperose skin.

SUNFLOWER

Forms Used: Ground seeds (sunflower seed meal)

Cosmetic Properties and Uses: Very rich in fatty acids, emollients, and beneficial nutrients. Meal makes a gentle, moisturizing scrub and mask base for normal-to-dry skin.

MAKING GRAIN, SEED, AND NUT MEALS

Almond Meal. To make ½ cup (125 ml) almond meal, grind (in 10-second pulses) approximately 50 large, raw almonds in a blender, coffee grinder, or food processor until the consistency is that of finely grated Parmesan cheese. Due to their high fat content, it's very easy to overblend almonds and end up with almond butter, especially if you use a small grinder that generates lots of heat. This is actually not a bad thing, as it is quite tasty and can be used just like peanut butter, but it's not the result you're after!

Flaxseed Meal. To make ½ cup (125 ml) flaxseed meal, blend a heaping ½ cup (125 ml) seeds in a blender, coffee grinder, or food processor until the consistency is that of coarse whole wheat flour.

Ground Oatmeal. To make ½ cup (125 ml) ground oatmeal, blend ¾ to 1 cup (180 to 250 ml) of regular or old-fashioned oats in a blender, coffee grinder, or food processor until the consistency is that of fine flour.

Sunflower Seed Meal. To make ½ cup (125 ml) sunflower seed meal, grind ¾ cup (180 ml) of large seeds (hulled) in a blender, coffee grinder, or food processor until the consistency is that of finely grated Parmesan cheese.

CLAY, SALT, THICKENERS, AND MISCELLANEOUS INGREDIENTS

This section outlines what I call "active ingredients," because they act as emulsifiers and binders, thickeners, humectants, preservatives, and pH balancers. These ingredients can be purchased through better health food and grocery stores, herb shops, and mail-order suppliers (see Resources).

BEESWAX
Form Used: Pure, unrefined, filtered or unfiltered beeswax
Cosmetic Properties and Uses: A thickener for making lip balms, salves, creams, and lotions. Purchase fresh from an apiary, if possible.

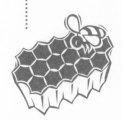

BORAX
Form Used: Crystalline powdered mineral salt
Cosmetic Properties and Uses: Can be bought in the laundry aisle of grocery stores. Acts as a binder and texturizer and, when combined with beeswax, oil, and water, makes a stable emulsion. Also acts as a whitener, mild antiseptic, and natural preservative.

CLAY, FRENCH GREEN
Form Used: Dried powder
Cosmetic Properties and Uses: A sage-green, highly mineralized clay, it's especially good for oily skin and for healing conditions that need drawing, astringency, sloughing, or circulation stimulation, such as acne, eczema, psoriasis, and devitalized, wrinkled skin.

CLAY, WHITE COSMETIC
Form Used: Dried powder
Cosmetic Properties and Uses: Preferred in facial care products for sensitive or normal-to-dry skin because of its gentleness. I use it when making masks and scrubs. Draws impurities from your skin, exfoliates, and remineralizes your complexion.

COCOA BUTTER
Form Used: Fatty cocoa wax or butter
Cosmetic Properties and Uses: Acts as a soothing emollient to sunburned and dry skin. Use in lip balms, creams, and lotions to soften the skin and thicken the product. Hardens in cold weather, but melts when applied to the skin.

GLYCERIN, VEGETABLE
Form Used: Clear, sweet thick liquid
Cosmetic Properties and Uses: Acts as a humectant, which means it draws moisture from the air to your skin. Use in lotions and creams for dry skin. Makes lip balms taste super sweet!

GRAPEFRUIT SEED EXTRACT
Common Names: Grapefruit extract, citrus seed extract, citrus extract
Form Used: Concentrated liquid extract
Cosmetic Properties and Uses: Used mainly as an astringent preservative and antimicrobial in the cosmetic industry. I add it to facial and body splashes, creams, and lotions to extend the shelf life of the product.

LANOLIN, ANHYDROUS
Form Used: Fat or wax from sheep's wool
Cosmetic Properties and Uses: An emollient that holds water on the skin. It absorbs water and is a terrific emulsifier for creams and lotions.
Contraindication: May be a potential allergen — do a patch test first.

SEA SALT
Form Used: Granular sea salt
Cosmetic Properties and Uses: Rich in minerals. Aids in healing oozing, itchy, rashy, inflamed skin. When added to bath water, sea salt can benefit skin afflicted with acne, eczema, psoriasis, poison plant rash, and other irritations.
Contraindication: Limit salt baths to 2 to 3 times per week as this mineral can be drying to the skin. Always follow a salt bath with an application of a good moisturizer.

VINEGAR, RAW APPLE CIDER
Form Used: Diluted vinegar
Cosmetic Properties and Uses: Softens and relieves itchy skin if added to bath water. I use it as a base for making herbal splashes and toners for all skin types. The natural fruit acids in vinegar act as a gentle exfoliant, leaving skin smooth and glowing. Restores normal pH to skin after cleansing.
Contraindication: May irritate sensitive or sunburned skin.

VITAMIN E (D-ALPHA TOCOPHEROL)
Form Used: Liquid capsule form
Cosmetic Properties and Uses: Acts as a natural preservative and antioxidant when added to creams, lotions, and base oils. Helps prevent rancidity. Reported to soften and gradually fade scar tissue. Fabulous relief for chapped lips and ragged cuticles.

WATER, DISTILLED
Form Used: Steam-distilled water
Cosmetic Properties and Uses: Used in making all cosmetic products that call for water or herb infusions. Will discourage premature mold growth in your cosmetics, which may occur if you use plain tap water.

WITCH HAZEL
Form Used: Liquid, water- and alcohol-based extract of witch hazel herb
Cosmetic Properties and Uses: Mild astringent. The ideal cleanser for minor cuts, scratches, and pimples. I use it as a facial splash base for normal-to-oily skin. The drugstore variety is fine.

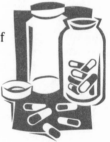

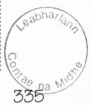

Bottles and Jars

Burch Bottle and Packaging
430 Hudson River Road
Waterford, NY 12188
(800) 903-2830
www.burchbottle.com

E.D. Luce Prescription
    Packaging
1600 East 29th Street
Signal Hill, CA 90806
(562) 997-9777
www.essentialsupplies.com

SKS Bottle and Packaging
3 Knabner Road
Mechanicville, NY 12118
(518) 899-7488
www.sks-bottle.com

Sunburst Bottle Company
5710 Auburn Boulevard #7
Sacramento, CA 95841
(916) 348-5576
www.sunburstbottle.com

Herb and Natural Product Suppliers

Aroma Vera
5310 Beethoven Street
Los Angeles, CA 90016
(800) 669-9514 ext. 4705
www.aromavera.com

Aromaland
1326 Rufina Circle
Sante Fe, NM 87507
(800) 933-5267
www.aromaland.com

Atlantic Spice Company
P.O. Box 205
North Truro, MA 02652
(800) 316-7965
www.altanticspice.com

Aura Cacia
P.O. Box 311
Norway, IA 52318
(800) 437-3301
www.frontiercoop.com

Avena Botanicals
219 Mill Street
Rockport, ME 04856
(207) 594-0694

Boericke & Tafel
2381 Circadian Way
Santa Rosa, CA 95407
(707) 571-8202

Brushy Mountain Bee Farm
610 Bethany Church Road
Moravian Falls, NC 28654
(800) BEESWAX

Dry Creek Herb Farm
14245 Edgehill Lane
Auburn, CA 95603
(530) 888-0889
www.drycreekherb farm.com

The Essential Oil Company
1719 SE Umatilla Street
Portland, OR 97202
(800) 729-5912
www.essentialoil.com

Fleur Aromatherapy
Langston Priory Mews
Kingham, Oxon
OX7 6UP, UK
+44 (0) 1608 659 909,
www.fleur.co.uk/front
    page.html

Frontier Co-op Herbs
P.O. Box 299
Norway, IA 52318
(800) 669-3275
www.frontiercoop.com

Janca's
456 East Juanita #7
Mesa, AZ 85204
(480) 497-9494
www.jancas.com

Jean's Greens
119 Sulphur Springs Road
Norway, NY 13416
(888) 845-8327
www.jeansgreens.com

Lavender Lane
7337 #1 Roseville Road
Sacramento, CA 95842
(888) 593-4400
www.lavenderlane.com

Liberty Natural Products
8120 SE Stark Street
Portland, OR 97215
(800) 289-8427
www.libertynatural.com

Motherlove Herbal
    Company
P.O. Box 101
LaPorte, CO 80535
(970) 493-2892
www.motherlove.com

Mountain Rose Herbs
85472 Dilley Lane
Eugene, OR 97405
(800) 879-3337
www.mountainrose
    herbs.com

Norfolk Lavender
777 New Durham Road
Edison, NJ 08817
(800) 886-0050
www.norfolklavender.com

Pacific Botanicals
4350 Fish Hatchery Road
Grants Pass, OR 97527
(541) 479-7777
www.pacificbotanicals.com

Pacific Institute of
    Aromatherapy
P.O. Box 6723
San Rafael, CA 94903
(415) 479-9120
www.pacificinstituteof
    aromatherapy.com

Penn Herb Company
10601 Decatur Road
Philadelphia, PA 19154
(800) 523-9971
www.pacificbotanicals.com

Sage Woman Herbs
406 S. 8th Street
Colorado Springs, CO
80905
(800) 350-3911
www.sagewomanherbs.com

September's Sun Herbal
Soap and Skin Care
Company
Stephanie Tourles, Owner
P.O. Box 772
W. Hyanisport, MA 02672
(508) 862-9955

Shirley Price
Aromatherapy Ltd.
Essentia House
Upper Bond Street
Hincley, Leicestershire
LE10 1RS, UK
+44 (0) 14 5561 5466
www.shirleyprice.com

Vermont Country Store
P.O. Box 3000
Manchester Center, VT
05255
(802) 362-2400
www.vermontcountry
store.com

**Education and
Associations**
The American Association
for Health Freedom
P.O. Box 458
Great Falls, VA 22066
(800) 230-2762
www.healthfreedom.net

American Association of
Naturopathic Physicians
8201 Greensboro Drive,
Suite 300
McLean, VA 22102
(877) 969-2267
www.naturopathic.org

American Botanical
Council
P.O. Box 144345
Austin, TX 78714
(512) 926-4900

American Herb Assoc.
P.O. Box 1673
Nevada City, CA 95959
(530) 265-9552

American Herbal Products
Association
8484 Georgia Ave., Ste. 370
Silver Spring, MD 20910
(301) 588-1174

American Herbalist's Guild
1931 Gaddis Road
Canton, GA 30115
(770) 751-6021
www.americanherbalist.com

Bio-Dynamic Farming and
Gardening Association
P.O. Box 29135
San Francisco, CA 94129
(888) 516-7797
www.biodynamics.com

Citizens for Health
5 Thomas Circle NW,
Suite 500
Washington, DC 20005
(202) 483-1652
www.citizens.org

Community Alliance with
Family Farmers
P.O. Box 363
Davis, CA 95617
(800) 852-3832

Herb Growing and
Marketing Network
P.O. Box 245
Silver Spring, PA 17575
(717) 393-3295
www.herbnet.com

Herb Research Foundation
1007 Pearl Street Ste. 200
Boulder, CO 80302
(303) 449-2265
www.herbs.org

International Federation
of Aromatherapists
182 Chiswick High Road
London W4 1PP, UK
+44 (0) 20 8742 2605
www.int-fed-aroma
therapy.co.uk

International Society of
Aromatherapists
ISPA House, 82 Ashby Rd.
Hinckley, Leicestershire
LE10 1SN, UK
+44 (0) 14 5563 7987,
www.the-ispa.org

Kerr Center for
Sustainable Agriculture
P.O. Box 588
Poteau, OK 74953
(918) 647-9123
www.kerrcenter.com

Lady Bird Johnson
Wildflower Center
4801 LaCrosse Avenue
Austin, TX 78739
(512) 292-4200
www.wildflower.org

Northeast Herbal Assoc.
P.O. Box 103
Manchaug, MA 01526
www.northeastherbal.org

United Plant Savers
P.O. Box 98
East Barre, VT 05649
www.plantsavers.org

**Periodicals
and Publications**
Acres USA: A Voice for
Eco-Agriculture
P.O. Box 91299
Austin, TX 78709
(800) 355-5313
www.acresusa.com

Dandelion Doings
Goosefoot Acres, Inc.
P.O. Box 18016
Cleveland, OH 44118
(216) 932-2145
www.edibleweeds.com

The Herb Companion
Interweave Press, Inc.
243 East Fourth Street
Loveland, CO 80537
(800) 272-2193
www.discoverherbs.com

INDEX